'In this book, Keith Oliver proves himself a worthy rival to his adversary, "Alzheimer's", to whom his annual letters are written. The book presents extracts from Keith's diary of the years since his diagnosis, interspersed with the annual letters – a combination of real-time and reflective writing that works beautifully. Add to this an interview about his writing, a play script and a postscript poem, and you have a rich mix about a full life which continues despite the best efforts of dementia. Keith does not hide his struggles and self-doubt but his appreciation for life and affection for others shine through, all delivered with a wry sense of humour.'

> – *Jan R. Oyebode, Professor of Dementia Care, Centre for*
> *Applied Dementia Studies, University of Bradford*

'I was so pleased to see that I made it into the list of "supporting cast" at the beginning of this book because Keith Oliver has certainly played a major part in helping me make sense of dementia. I have worked as a clinician and an academic in dementia care for over 30 years but this book makes sense of dementia in the context of a life well lived. Because of Keith I don't fear getting dementia as much. I don't want the little memory slips I experience to be early signs of dementia but, if they are, reading how Keith has coped makes me think maybe I could too. I highly recommend this book to all involved in supporting people diagnosed with dementia as well as those directly affected.'

> – *Professor Dawn Brooker PhD CPsychol (clin) AFBPsS, Director of*
> *the Association for Dementia Studies at University of Worcester*

'What a delightful and uniquely written insight into dementia by Keith Oliver, highlighting it is possible to live more positively with dementia than everyone once thought. Through his diary, which at times felt like being "on the inside" of a play, we have been given a rich and meaningful view of his life, and of dementia. I highly recommend Keith's book, including suggesting it is added to your local library collection.'

> – *Kate Swaffer, Chair, CEO and Co-founder of Dementia Alliance*
> *International, Disability Rights Activist and author*

'In a novel diary format, Keith records the daily ups and downs of his struggle dementia. His honesty and courage is refreshing and insightful, throughou enriching and powerful book, which needs to be read by all people seeking a diag and families, as well as service providers and researchers.'

> – *Dr Christine Bryden, author and person living with dem*

'From quiet beginnings of disbelief at the diagnosis to the loud voice of an activist. Keith's diaries show how with the love and support of those around you, the darkness of a diagnosis can turn into the sunlight of new beginnings even with dementia in tow.'
– *Wendy Mitchell, author of Sunday Times Bestseller* Somebody I Used to Know

'Readers, draw strength, inspiration and hope from *Dear Alzheimer's*. Keith's fortitude, determination and wisdom as he adapts to life with young onset dementia are engagingly expressed throughout this well-penned book. It is these qualities, together with Keith's honesty, judgement and humour, that have brought so much of value to our charity, YoungDementia UK and to the Young Dementia Network through our association with each other. Long may it continue.'
– *Tessa Gutteridge, Director of YoungDementia UK*
and Chair of Young Dementia Network

'A candid, moving account from a courageous man – this book gives thoughtful and at times heart-breaking insight into living with dementia.'
– *Victoria Derbyshire, award-winning journalist and broadcaster*

'What a journal of times before, during and since diagnosis! It also gives me an insight into some of my own lapses of timeline and "not quite as I remember it" events. I feel such solidarity with Keith and his wife.'
– *Jayne Goodrick, carer, advocate, friend*

'I begin writing this endorsement, which I am humbled and honoured to do, with a slightly heavy heart, because the more I read, the more my own life with dementia resonated through Keith's writings. This is a really honest and deep look into his life, through his eyes, and the trials and tribulations are going to inspire everyone who reads, and give those living with a dementia diagnosis, "permission to carry on living their lives, by making adaptations and understanding what they are now living with". Well done to my now very good friend.'
– *Chris Roberts, person living with and advocating*
for all those affected by dementia

DEAR ALZHEIMER'S

of related interest

Will I Still Be Me?
Finding a Continuing Sense of Self in the Lived Experience of Dementia
Christine Bryden
ISBN 978 1 78592 555 9
eISBN 978 1 78450 950 7

What the Hell Happened to My Brain?
Living Beyond Dementia
Kate Swaffer
ISBN 978 1 84905 608 3
eISBN 978 1 78450 073 3

A Pocket Guide to Understanding Alzheimer's Disease and Other Dementias, Second Edition
Dr James Warner and Dr Nori Graham
ISBN 978 1 78592 458 3
eISBN 978 1 78450 835 7

Dancing with Dementia
My Story of Living Positively with Dementia
Christine Bryden
ISBN 978 1 84310 332 5
eISBN 978 1 84642 095 5

Dear Alzheimer's

A Diary of
Living with Dementia

Keith Oliver

Forewords by Carey Mulligan and
Professor Linda Clare and Rachael Litherland

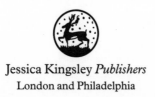

Jessica Kingsley *Publishers*
London and Philadelphia

Half of the royalties from the sale of this book will go to supporting Young Dementia UK.

The flower image used on title pages is adapted from Kitwood, T. (2019) *Dementia Reconsidered Revisited: The Person Still Comes First* (ed. Dawn Brooker). London: Open University Press.

First published in 2019
by Jessica Kingsley Publishers
73 Collier Street
London N1 9BE, UK
and
400 Market Street, Suite 400
Philadelphia, PA 19106, USA

www.jkp.com

Library of Congress Cataloging in Publication Data
A CIP catalog record for this book is available from the Library of Congress

British Library Cataloguing in Publication Data
A CIP catalogue record for this book is available from the British Library

ISBN 978 1 78592 503 0
eISBN 978 1 78450 898 2

Printed and bound in Great Britain

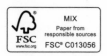

Whilst writing this book, others who live every day with young onset dementia have never been far from my thoughts. I hope that by reading this book you gain some strength and positivity to see that it is possible to live a full and active life beyond the diagnosis.

In my view, to do this love and support are essential, and I have been lucky to have received both in larger quantities than I could expect or deserve. Consequently I dedicate my book to all those living with young onset dementia or caring for us as loved ones or professionals.

Thank you – this one is for all of you.

Contents

Foreword

Carey Mulligan, *Alzheimer's Society's UK Global*
Dementia Friends Ambassador

I've had the privilege of meeting Keith on a number of occasions when we carry out our respective roles as Alzheimer's Society Ambassadors.

I have always been struck by his eloquence, compassion and quiet yet steely determination in tackling his diagnosis and uniting others against dementia. This book tells the story of the extraordinary commitment Keith shows every day in changing people's perceptions of dementia and his role in fighting for the rights of all those living with the condition, now and in the future.

Reading Keith's words highlights just how active and engaged he is in all his campaigning and the contribution he and others make to create lasting change. He paints a vivid picture of the moment he and his wife, Rosemary, were told of his diagnosis, the courage in not just accepting it themselves, but the additional struggles they faced in telling others the devastating news and having to give up his job as a much respected Headteacher. Their worlds were turned upside down but Keith has now turned this around into being an ardent activist for change.

Keith is an inspiration certainly to me, and I think should be to us all.

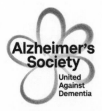

Foreword

Professor Linda Clare *and* **Rachael Litherland**

Keith, as he himself tells 'Dear Alzheimer's' in this book, will never be defined by dementia. The qualities that do define him include his wisdom, his care for others, his generosity, his openness and his readiness to share his experience – in short, his personhood.

Although he is not defined by dementia, he is one of those rare people who helps us understand, from the inside, what it is really like to live with the condition. For both of us, his contribution to our work has been exceptional and greatly valued. As a prominent dementia activist, his perspective has informed both our research and many innovative and creative projects aimed at changing and improving life for people affected by dementia.

Following his diagnosis several years ago, his willingness to share his journey of adjustment to life with dementia has helped many people, showing that dementia is life-changing, not life-ending. He embodies a positive and constructive approach to trying to live with this life-changing condition, supported and encouraged by his wife Rosemary.

In this book he grapples with his thoughts and feelings about dementia and takes us on a new journey challenging accepted ways of viewing the condition. He shares examples of how continuing to engage with life around you can help maintain a sense of purpose and find new solutions to some of the dilemmas of everyday life with dementia. This is an insightful account of how one person deals with what dementia throws at you day by day. Everyone's path with dementia is different, but Keith's experience will inspire and enable others to find their own way of tackling life with dementia.

Taking a different approach to previous books, Keith draws on his diaries, journals and extensive notes made since receiving his diagnosis to construct a unique and personal account. This is a valuable addition to the growing body of literature describing from an individual perspective what it is like to live with dementia.

Through our ongoing work with Keith, not only has our work benefited, but our own lives have been enriched and our understanding deepened. IDEAL (Improving the Experience of Dementia and Enhancing Active Life) programme advisory group meetings would not be the same without Keith there to keep us on track with the agenda! We look forward to continuing fruitful collaborations.

Acknowledgements

I refer often in my life and in this book to the 'Kitwood flower', and it is deliberate that each chapter carries an element which Tom Kitwood, a pioneer in the field of dementia care, placed in the petals and centre of the flower that he devised. For me, and for Kitwood, at the centre of the 'flower' is love, love for my family and for the friends who have helped and supported me since I was given the diagnosis of Alzheimer's disease.

Always first and foremost with any acknowledgement of love and support is Rosemary, without whom I certainly would not be here today. Every page of this book has within it her presence. She was the first reader of the draft manuscript and as always gave me constructive suggestions and encouragement to persevere. Next, although not prominently written about, are my family, who remain closest to my heart and mind – it is thanks to Gareth, Karon, James, Byron, Rhian and William that 'the fog' is pushed away, and 'the sun' brought in.

Prior to summer 2017 I did not know Andrew James, senior commissioning editor at Jessica Kingsley Publishing. Now I feel truly blessed that Andrew came into my world when totally out of the blue he contacted me to invite discussion about a possible book. Andrew has been a really true friend and ally throughout this project. He is always supportive, encouraging, calm and absolutely open to working together on our collaboration. Thank you Andrew, I hope our friendship will last well beyond this book.

I always have been most at ease with the support of a team alongside me, and this book is another example of this being the case. First and foremost, one central person in my story is Reinhard Guss. 'Dankeschön Reinhard mein Kamerad. Freundschaft hat keine Grenzen' (*Thank you very much Reinhard my comrade. Friendship has no boundaries*). Moving on to five friends whose commitment has far exceeded anything I could have hoped for or expected: Nicki Griffiths, Lewis Slade, Liz Jennings, April Doyle and Dr Jocelyne Kenny have brought to life attachment, comfort, identity, occupation, inclusion and – yes – love through our friendship. Thank you, I am so lucky to know you all and I treasure and value our friendship.

A number of students on placement with the NHS have brought far more than positive support into my world, as the reader, I hope, can appreciate through this book; indeed, during the writing of the book Darshi Mano, Andrew Coleman and Abi Hassan brought alongside skill and diligence such wide-eyed enthusiasm, which was infectious and energising. As you move into professional roles, please do your best to retain this.

I often say the best thing that has happened to me since being diagnosed is the people who have come into my life, and many of them are featured in this book. I would like to express special thanks to Professor Linda Clare and Rachael Litherland for kindly agreeing to write the foreword to this book, to Jen Holland for her friendship and photographic skills and to Tessa Gutteridge, CEO of Young Dementia UK, for all she and the charity she leads do to help people affected by young onset dementia and for supporting me in championing this book. I am thrilled that half of the royalties will benefit Young Dementia UK.

Everyone mentioned in *Dear Alzheimer's* deserves my sincerest thanks, and please do not feel if you are excluded from these acknowledgements that I value your support any less, because I do not. Many of you have stayed in my life over the past eight years and for this I am extremely grateful.

Keith Oliver
Canterbury 2018

Dear Alzheimer's letters

Dear reader

I feel I am well placed to recognise and appreciate the importance attached to the kind, considerate and non-judgemental support of friends, and I hope that this is reflected in the letter sections of my book. The concept began through such a friendship with Eric Harmer and Jen Holland, both of whom encouraged me to read and give thought to the writings of C.S. Lewis, and introducing me to his book *The Screwtape Letters*. This is in essence an ironic portrayal of human life from the point of view of Screwtape, an apprentice nephew of the devil. Associated with this, whilst the letters may be seen constructively by some as epistolary, this was not my intention.

Initially I took this idea and tried to write letters from my Alzheimer's to me, or anyone sharing their brain with, as Terry Pratchett termed it, 'this wretched embuggerance'. The resulting initial letter was, though, so depressing and dark that I felt the reader would be too alarmed by the content. So, after giving it some considerable further thought, I decided to turn the concept on its head and write from myself to the dark beast that dwells in my brain which at times I humanise as 'Dr Alzheimer'. This in turn morphed slightly, partly out of respect to Dr Alois Alzheimer whose name is now forever associated with this disease, into letters to 'dear Alzheimer's'.

I would not wish you, the reader, to think that I feel there is anything 'dear' about Alzheimer's, or communicating with one's Alzheimer's, but I ask that you consider this on two levels: first, the letters are actually written to myself, and are designed to help con-firm that I am not easily giving in to the clutches of the disease, and second, the use of the word 'dear' is meant to convey a sense of irony and sarcasm which I think is further endorsed in the way I have signed off and closed each letter.

Whilst there is an element of creativity and originality in the letters, they are not to be read as fiction: they are in my mind factual and truthful, based upon notes taken from my diaries and journals, and should be read alongside the larger sections of the book, which is diary based and upon which the letters are closely drawn.

So, dear reader, and this time the sentiment is sincere and genuine, I hope that with this in mind you like what I have attempted to convey, and that irrespective of where you are coming from to my book you can take something from this.

Many thanks and very best wishes

Keith

Supporting cast in order of appearance of people who appear more than once

Rosemary Oliver – My wife and supporter

Jim Reed – BBC reporter on the *Victoria Derbyshire* show

Dr Aston – Consultant psychiatrist, Kent and Medway Partnership Trust (KMPT)

Andrew Coleman – Kent University placement student, KMPT

Darshi Mano – Kent University placement student, KMPT

Christopher Devas – Person living with dementia

Alec Murrell – Deputy head and acting head at Blean Primary School

Chi Chi Nwanoku – Musician

Kim – Secretary to the neurologists

Pam Godden – Bursar at Blean Primary School

Dr Christian Farthing – Spinal specialist, BodyWell, Canterbury

Dr Nori Graham – Psychiatrist and author

Dr James Warner – Psychiatrist and author

Annette Kelly – HR manager at Kent County Council

Alan and Glenys Brokenshire – Aussie friends

John Davies – Retired caretaker, Blean Primary School, now friend

Jean Markham – John's partner

James – Son

Jane and Ian Harris – Cousin and her husband

Maisie Snell – Auntie

Lynne Lawrence – My successor at Blean Primary School

Dr Elizabeth Field – Clinical psychologist, KMPT

Jouko Koecher – Assistant psychologist, KMPT

Tom Hunt – Teacher at Blean Primary School

Sinead McGettrick – Admiral Nurse (specialist dementia nurse)

Gerry Warren – Senior reporter at the *Kentish Gazette* newspaper

Dr Richard Brown – Consultant psychiatrist, KMPT

Reinhard Guss – Consultant clinical psychologist, KMPT

Judy Ayris – Age UK, Canterbury

Clive Close – Head teacher, Wincheap Primary School

Jean and Andy Robinson – Next-door neighbours

Daren Kerle – Community librarian, Kent County Council

Dr Penny Hibberd – Director, Dementia Centre, Canterbury Christ Church University

Celia Rigden – Fellow Forget Me Nots member

Gareth – Eldest son

Dominic McCully – Solicitor

Ian Asquith – Kent University placement student, KMPT

Matt Murray – Manager, Alzheimer's Society Research Network

Jan and Wayne Darling – Aussie friends

Julie and Paul Reece – Aussie friends

Bev and John Endersbee – Aussie friends

Tom Kitwood – Author and legend

Dr Nick Branch – Son-in-law

Dr Barbara Beats – Consultant psychiatrist, KMPT

Gaynor Smith – User involvement manager, Alzheimer's Society

Sarah Tilsed – Dementia Action Alliance

Professor Jan Dewing – Director, Dementia Centre, Canterbury Christ Church University

Pat Chung – Head of occupational therapy studies, Canterbury Christ Church University

Larry Gardiner – Fellow activist living with dementia

Mycal Miller – Film maker

Julia Burton-Jones – Dementia UK/ Dementia Pathfinders

Heather Rolfe – Kent University placement student, KMPT

Peter Ashley – Fellow activist living with dementia

Eric Bogle – Singer-songwriter

Tanya Clover – Independent dementia consultant

Christine Bryden – Fellow activist living with dementia

Richard Taylor – Fellow activist living with dementia

Kate Swaffer – Fellow activist living with dementia

David Cameron – UK Prime Minister

Professor Dawn Brooker – Director of the Association of Dementia Studies, Worcester University

April Doyle – Friend, writing tutor, project lead administrator, Community Arts and Education Programme, Canterbury Christ Church University

Alison Culverwell – Consultant clinical psychologist, KMPT

Nada Savitch – Director, Innovations in Dementia

Rachael Litherland – Director, Innovations in Dementia

Steve Milton – Director, Innovations in Dementia

Carey Mulligan – Actor, Alzheimer's Society ambassador

Jane Cotton – Senior celebrity liaison officer, Alzheimer's Society

Professor Craig Ritchie – Psychiatrist, researcher

Melvyn Brooks – Fellow Forget Me Nots member

Jan Brooks – Melvyn's wife

Lewis Slade – Kent University placement student, KMPT

Christian Bakker – Healthcare Psychologist and researcher, Radboud Nijmegen University

Sarah Ghani – Clinical psychologist

Alex Bone – Kent University placement student, KMPT

Janet Lloyd – Patient, Public and Community Involvement (PPCI) manager, KMPT

Jon Parsons – Director, KMPT

Sophie Razzel – Kent University placement student, KMPT

Charley Massingham – Kent University placement student, KMPT

Jen Holland (née Russell) – Friend/ Kent University placement student, KMPT

Carolina – Fellow Forget Me Nots member

Kim Robinson – Lecturer, Kent University

Angela Rippon – TV presenter, Alzheimer's Society ambassador

Jocelyne Kenny – Trainee psychologist, KMPT

Liz Jennings – Friend and co-leader of projects with me

Janet Baylis – Manager, Alzheimer's Society Knowledge Centre

Rachel Thompson – Dementia project leader at the Royal College of Nursing

Chris Norris – Forget Me Nots member and fellow KMPT envoy

Toby Williamson – Mental Health Foundation coordinator of the Dementia Truth Inquiry

Dr Daphne Wallace – Fellow activist living with dementia, co-chair of the Dementia Truth Inquiry

Hellen Riley – Aussie friend

Lisa Bogue – Engagement and participation officer, Alzheimer's Society

Winifred Robinson – Presenter on BBC Radio 4's *You and Yours*

Angeliki Argyriou – Assistant psychologist, KMPT

Dr Noel Collins – Consultant psychiatrist

Barbara and Michael Field – sister-in-law and brother-in-law

Katie Bennett – Media officer, Alzheimer's Society

Amy Merritt (née Morrish) – Friend and ex-primary school pupil

Chris Ryan – Fellow Forget Me Nots member

Jess Amos – Kent University placement student, KMPT

Professor Alistair Burns – Professor of old age psychiatry, National Clinical Director for Dementia, NHS England

Ingrid Tamuyeye – Kent University placement student, KMPT

Sumita Chauhan – Sculptural artist/ PhD student, Kent University

Chris Roberts – Fellow activist living with dementia

Jayne Roberts – Chris's wife

Wendy Mitchell – Fellow activist living with dementia

Jane Roberts – Psychotherapist, KMPT

Leonard Cohen – Singer-songwriter

Professor Graham Stokes – BUPA, co-chair of the Dementia Truth Inquiry

Veronica Devas – Christopher Devas's wife and carer

Ellie Anslow – Kent University placement student, KMPT

Richard Madeley – TV and radio presenter, writer of foreword to *Walk the Walk, Talk the Talk* and Alzheimer's Society supporter

Eric Harmer – Friend

Claire Thorpe – Project support officer, Alzheimer's Society

Adrian Taylor ('Tats') and Anne Hobbs – Friends

Frances James – Placement and volunteer coordinator, School of Psychology, Kent University

Dr Yvette Kusel – Clinical psychologist, KMPT

Peter Watson – Carer, fellow member of Young Onset Network steering group

Nicki Chisnall – Kent University placement student, KMPT

Tricia Fincher – Kent Libraries community officer – older people

Kate Comfort (née Taylor) – Dementia support worker, Alzheimer's Society

Dr Alex Hillman – Cardiff University researcher on IDEAL project

Briony Russell – Kent University placement student, KMPT

Vishy – Kent University placement student, KMPT

Michael Blackburn – Kent University placement student, KMPT

Kai Pang – Kent University placement student, KMPT

Nicky Thompson – Community development officer, Canterbury City Council

Byron – Grandson

Rhian – Granddaughter

William – Grandson

Karon – Daughter

Tommy Dunne – Fellow activist living with dementia

Claire Garley – Engagement and participation officer, Alzheimer's Society

Paul Simon – Singer-songwriter

Rachel Niblock – Dementia Engagement and Empowerment Project (DEEP), Innovations in Dementia

Jo Brand – Comedian, TV celebrity and writer of foreword to *Welcome to Our World*

Bill Turnbull – BBC TV presenter and Alzheimer's Society supporter

Hilary Doxford – Fellow activist living with dementia

Polly Yoncheva – Canterbury Christ Church University placement student, KMPT

Kristina Sigetova – Kent University placement student, KMPT

Carol Fordyce – Fellow Forget Me Nots member

Lorraine Brown – Fellow activist living with dementia

Philly Hare – DEEP, Innovations in Dementia

Sammi Bellamy – Canterbury Christ Church University placement student, KMPT

Celina Stephanie – Kent University placement student, KMPT

Charles Ryan – Fellow Forget Me Nots member

Pauline Ryan – Charles's wife and carer

Elizabeth Oliver – Engagement and participation officer, Alzheimer's Society

Abi Hassan – Canterbury Christ Church University placement student, KMPT

Donna Chadwick – National Development Manager, Young Dementia Network

Dr Doug Brown – Director of research, Alzheimer's Society

Professor Peter Mittler – Fellow activist living with dementia

Dr Catherine Quinn – Senior research fellow, Exeter University

Andrew James – Senior commissioning editor, Jessica Kingsley Publishers

Sabrina Jantuah – Engagement and participation officer, Alzheimer's Society

Nicki Griffiths – a friend

Rachel Hutchings – Policy officer, Alzheimer's Society

Phil Freeman – Dementia Action Alliance

Jo Vidal – Clinical psychologist, KMPT

Dr Rebecca Reed – Lead clinical psychologist for complex care and dementia, Cornwall Partnership NHS Foundation Trust

Alan Stumpenhuson-Payne – MA student connected to Dreams and Visions project

Thank you everyone for being alongside me from there to here, and hopefully beyond.

Introduction

4th January 2018 – Canterbury

As I sit in my armchair looking around my lounge at what has been today a mock-up, busy film studio, I am now left on my own with a coffee kindly made for me by Rosemary before she headed out ten minutes ago to the supermarket, and my mind is racing as it seeks to make sense of what thoughts, views and memories have been explored during the day.

Jim Reed, a reporter from the BBC's *Victoria Derbyshire* show, has left a few minutes ago after six hours of filming at my house for a forthcoming edition of the programme which will update viewers on my story and that of Wendy and Christopher Devas, which was previously broadcast in April 2015. Like some others I have been lucky to work with since being diagnosed, Jim cares about both his work and those whose stories he seeks to tell fairly, honestly and compassionately, and although I am already struggling to remember what we discussed, and what he filmed, I am left with a sense of today being a 'sunny' or good day. This experience has caused me to reflect upon the last seven years, as many of his questions focused upon changes around looking both backwards and forwards – a little like Janus, the two-headed Roman god who looked back at the old year and forward towards the new.

I am unsure what I would have thought back in January 2010 had someone told me then that a few months later I would be diagnosed with a disease which is reported to be the most feared amongst the over-45 age group and the largest cause of death now in this country. The words of Dr Aston, my initial consultant psychiatrist, are running through my mind as I write this. I asked her how long I would have until I was a typical person with dementia. Whatever that meant. She shrugged and said, 'I don't know. Six months? Six years?' She wouldn't go beyond that. Here I am, seven years later being filmed by the BBC. Am I the same person? How have I changed? I look in the mirror and I see a reflection of myself. I read what I have written. I watch myself on film. Whilst the images are clear, the memories are not. How do I see myself? How do people see me? Some have known me from before 2010, others have come into my life since.

My book tells this narrative with a focus on the past seven or eight years. I have opened my diaries and journals to you, the reader, as, indeed, I have opened my world for you to visit the foggy recesses of my mind. My diary remains as it always has been, a vital planning aid looking forward to forthcoming events and commitments, but has also increasingly served as a substitute hippocampus: logging and beginning the process of making sense of and then placing thoughts, feelings and conversations in an increasingly flawed filing system of my brain. I need to strive to be able to thrive, and I demand an awful lot of myself, leaning heavily on my diary and journal notes which I read, check, re-read, check and read again. My memory was very good until my early 50s. My father used to say, 'Keith has a photogenic memory'; he was nearly right! This was the case even during my hazy days as a student, this time caused by cramming beer, chips and lecture content into what was a reasonably good body and mind.

My appearance is largely the same, and when I am remembering to do my balance exercise my walk seems the same. Whilst words sometimes confound me, my voice remains unchanged; despite all of this I feel fundamentally different, and central to this is that my thinking is now almost always emotionally dominated. I hope this book gives the reader insight into the world of a person with dementia, how I strive to live as well as possible, and how this journey has thus far taken me on many ups and downs.

Not long ago, I was a head teacher managing a 460-pupil school with 45 staff and an annual budget in excess of £1.3 million with a new £100,000 building project. In addition, I was supporting a range of other Canterbury schools in my advisor role, and studying for a master's degree at a local university. I went from this to doing nothing, following which I was faced with trying to re-establish myself within my new life by dealing with these changes.

Although I am no longer functioning as a professional teacher, there is a continuing thread to my story. It's been said of me that, once a teacher, always a teacher. In part this is told through intergenerational projects which have always been important to me. I enjoyed working with children, supporting young enthusiastic newly qualified teachers, and serving on interview panels at the local university to help select the next intake beginning their journey into the most honourable profession of teaching. This has continued through to writing this introduction with the patient support of Andrew and Darshi, two University of Kent students on placement with Kent and Medway Partnership Trust (KMPT).

Indeed one door closing; one door opening.

2010

—

'One door closes, one door opens'

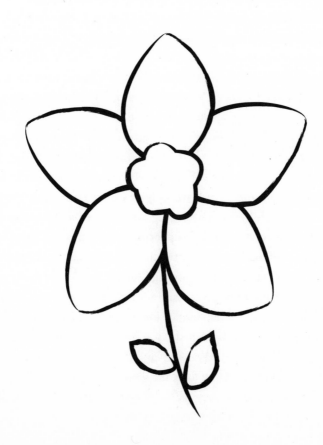

10th February – On a train from Maidstone

On crisp, bright days such as today travelling through the Weald of Kent, I feel blessed to live in this corner of our country. Alongside this sense of relaxation after a day at the Maidstone office, I am though troubled by uncertainty, which puzzles me as it is for me an unusual experience. Decision making has come relatively easily to me over the years, and now I am uncertain about my professional future. Do I return to my school headship after a two-year secondment as an education advisor, or do I resign from school and take the offer of a new role with the Local Authority Advisory Service? I value this time to think on the train, time to ponder my future and then over the next few days to talk to those closest to me personally and professionally.

15th February – Canterbury

Working from home for the past two years and visiting schools in and around Canterbury has been a very stimulating experience after 32 wonderful years working in schools. Most of the time I have enjoyed this new working pattern and the freedom and responsibility associated with this. Also, each month, I go to Maidstone for meetings with the Primary Excellence Project, for which I act as an advisor. My role has been to advise the 23 primary schools in Canterbury. I have thrived on the challenges that the role has presented through various projects, and have found working with head teachers to usually be both rewarding and stimulating. I have particularly enjoyed working with the newly qualified teachers who are the next generation of professionals who I hope can be inspired to take up the baton of creative, child-centred learning, and despite the stresses associated with Ofsted inspections which I supported schools through alongside the negativity around local government politics which I hated, I hope that the schools recognise my role in supporting them.

The past year has been particularly rewarding because our Partnership (which is the word for the supposedly joined-up local government services provided for children) has been the second most improved of all the 23 across Kent at Key Stage 2. Whilst plaudits for this have been nice, it is really due to the hard work put in by the schools themselves. All that I have needed to do is to provide some personal and professional encouragement, facilitation and steering, and this has been very enjoyable to do whilst hopefully bringing some benefit to the schools, and most importantly to the children the schools are serving.

23rd February – Maidstone

On the train today to my monthly meeting of the Primary Excellence Project (PEP) team I reflected upon some of the projects I have led over the past two years, and whilst I have felt a bit 'off' mentally recently, and had a fall or two which I do not understand, my physical health feels fine. I try and focus upon my job and four of the big projects for Canterbury area primary schools which I have led; these are a £26,000 project to develop better music education; £25,000 to develop modern foreign languages – largely though not exclusively French; a £2500 grant to support me in helping advanced skilled teachers, who in the past had no support, to develop writing with our 10/11-year-olds; and £6000 to treat head teachers and deputies with the respect they deserve with fit-for-purpose meetings in a venue which is conducive to collaborative working. Looking at this list of key projects, I do feel I have given the role my 'best shot' and Canterbury primary schools are, I hope, better placed than they were two years ago to deliver for our children.

After devoting a lot of thought to my future I am looking forward to a number more years back at my school to continue to try and make a difference for those children in my care. Key influences in my decision making include wanting to lead and teach and not to judge; to nurture and not to criticise; to create and not dismantle; and to encourage and not demean in an environment over which I and similar-minded colleagues at least have some control over.

1st March – Maidstone

Sitting in a meeting room at the education office, thinking about the past two years on secondment, and looking forward, now having made my mind up, to returning to school. The workshop that I am listening to is frustratingly like a number of these: 80 per cent bullshit, 20 per cent a waste of time. The guy delivering today even used last year's figures for this year's graphs. Inexcusable. Really good meetings stand out in my memory, but there are many like this one.

3rd March – Canterbury

I've been giving a lot of thought to returning to school, and to my resignation from the PEP team. I am looking forward to going back to school. I have enjoyed the PEP job, but it's also involved a lot of politics and a lot of travel, and I do miss my school – the familiarity and the sense of satisfaction of working in my own school. I also miss my colleagues and most of all I miss the children, so all of this is a driver towards encouraging me to go back.

I've explained this to Ruth, who has been my manager during most of the secondment, and she understands, whilst quietly encouraging me to make the decision to stay on as an advisor. I have also explained it to Alec, who as the acting head, and my deputy, needed to know pretty soon, so that he could organise what he wished to do: whether he wished to return to being a deputy, or whether he wanted to choose to benefit from the two years of being an acting head to seek a substantive post elsewhere.

15th March – Canterbury

I decided to see the GP, as I have been concerned about my health recently – largely because of my balance. I feel as though I am on a ship in rough seas, and maybe I've got an ear infection, so I have finally decided to get this checked out, and hopefully antibiotics will help. Having had a couple of years of waterworks infections and sinus infections, I guess this time I'm being confronted with an ear infection, and hope medication will sort the problem.

It is now 6 p.m. I have seen the GP, and she confirmed that there was no obvious infection in my ears, but gave me antibiotics just in case. She tested my balance, which wasn't at all good, and told me to come back in two weeks if there's no improvement.

29th March – Canterbury

Back to the GP – there's been no improvement, and I've had another fall. I still feel as though I'm on a ship.

Last time I saw a different GP, today I saw my usual GP, and he gave me some more tests, and checked my balance by asking me to stand on one leg and to walk heel to toe – I never realised how really hard this is! He patiently asked me some questions about how my concentration was and he spoke to Rosemary with me. The outcome was that he has decided to send me for a brain scan. Which is interesting. I haven't got a clue why he's sending me for this. He didn't say.

The location of the falls has been puzzling. I've fallen twice at home, and once in a bookshop in town. And I've started to use a stick discreetly. I don't like using it, but it does help me with my balance. I don't use it when I'm at work as I do not want to alarm anyone or draw attention to my health. The time I find it most helpful is if I go for a walk somewhere, maybe over the fields, or if I go to the shop; I'll carry it in my bag and use it if I need it.

30th March – Canterbury

I am attending my regular sessions for my master's course at Canterbury Christ Church University. There's about 12 of us: 11 secondary school teachers and deputies, and myself as the sole primary school member of the group. I am about one year into the course, and it's going very well. The assignments are both stimulating and challenging, and my results are good, with marks of 62 per cent and 65 per cent, which is in line with a good pass at MA level. I enjoy the stimulation of the course although I am now finding it quite tiring, as it comes after a day at work on a Tuesday evening from 6.30 to 8.30, so it does make a long day. I am feeling a bit frustrated with myself as I have been feeling extra tired recently, and struggling a little with my concentration, and I have noticed things have not been going into the old grey matter as readily as they did previously. However, it's not given me any great cause for concern. I guess I'm just not as young as I used to be! I've not spoken about this to anybody, just noted it in my diary really. I am trying to remain focused and positive by looking forward to the next session in two weeks' time. The MA is focused upon education leadership, and my next assignment is to focus on leadership of the teaching assistants because that's something that will be of real importance to the school when I return to Blean after Easter.

1st April – Maidstone

The final meeting with the PEP team, my last day as an advisor for Canterbury primary schools. I had a lovely send-off from colleagues, and some really touching cards and messages from head teachers in the Canterbury area. It appears as though they have enjoyed working with me in this role, remembering that I've been a head teacher with them for nine years previously, so I knew most of them as colleagues. It was an interesting transition, from being a colleague to being an advisor. I guess some would find that difficult, but I actually found it quite easy. Boundaries were easy to secure and build upon, while not letting them get in the way of the cooperation and collaboration between us.

Heading back home tonight on the train, I am now feeling at ease with the situation, looking forward to an Easter break, and then starting back at Blean again. During the secondment I have returned to Blean at least once a month, sometimes more often than that. Not so frequently that Alec thought I was breathing down his neck, but enough to keep an eye on the school alongside meeting with key members of staff. The school was run well over the two years, and some of the changes Alec brought in I'd wish to maintain, whilst others I'd wish to revert back to as they were in 2008 when I temporarily handed over the reins, which I am now very excited to be taking up again after the Easter break.

12th April – Canterbury

The date for the scan has now come through, and I am going off to Kent and Canterbury hospital today to have an MRI (magnetic resonance imaging) brain scan.

It's now the afternoon, and I've returned from the hospital, having had the brain scan. Interesting experience – I didn't find it too stressful. I don't really suffer with claustrophobia, so being enclosed inside the scanner for 45 minutes with some nice music playing, and able to give some thought to going back to school, was actually quite helpful and therapeutic.

I wouldn't say I enjoyed it, but it wasn't that bad at all. Not as bad as I expected. Although I really don't know why they're scanning me, and what it's all about. Certainly, the appointment came through very quickly – within two weeks!

13th April – Blean, Canterbury

In school today, to meet with Alec and the other deputies to do a handover meeting, and to discuss in greater detail what we have covered in the last few months in the build-up to my return.

All seems to be very smooth and orderly, and it's looking as though Alec is contemplating very seriously moving onto a headship. I'll do all I can to support him because I feel he's ready, and will hopefully do a really good job at whatever school he goes to.

19th April – Canterbury

After a restful Easter holiday I feel energised and I am looking forward to and excited about my return to school. Today, we've got a staff development day, and I've booked Howfield Manor, a pleasant venue on the outskirts of Canterbury set in lovely grounds, to re-establish myself as head, and to give staff the chance to have a really positive and productive day together. We are going to cover lots of issues during the day around creative schools and children's learning, alongside planning for the forthcoming term together. A full day supported by a convivial meal together.

Back to my diary at the end of the day, having returned home feeling very tired, but energised by what we are hoping to achieve this term, this year and beyond, as I seek to move the school forward as the head, with a really very good team of staff alongside me. After many disturbed nights thinking about my return to school I know I will sleep well tonight.

20th April – Canterbury

I had a concerned call today from the GP slightly out of the blue. He told me to listen carefully to the neurologist at the forthcoming appointment, and then phone him back. Well, I don't really understand this. I have an appointment with the neurologist in two days' time. Surely the GP phone call and the appointment are linked, but whether it was fear or being caught off guard I didn't ask my GP any questions, which is not like me. I checked the appointment letter, signed by a neurologist named Dr Redmond. I suppose what I'll have to do is exactly as the GP said and take notes, which is something I have always done to an extent, although my memory has usually been pretty reliable. I am reassured also because Rosemary will be with me. Understandably Rosemary thought it unlike me that I hadn't sought more information from the GP, and all I could say was that we'll just have to see how we go.

22nd April – Canterbury

Had a phone call from the hospital today, from the secretary of Dr Redmond, to apologise, and say that my appointment has been cancelled as he is abroad stuck in the US by the volcanic dust cloud which is causing an enormous disruption to travel. The media are currently full of the story, and newsreaders are making a valiant attempt to pronounce the previously obscure volcano Eyjafjallajökull. It causes me to reflect that when you see these things on the news, you do not always realise the impact they may have on you personally.

So now I've been told to await an alternative appointment. It may be with Dr Redmond, or it may be with one of his colleagues.

23rd April – Blean

We had a really interesting visitor today at school, a lady called Chi Chi Nwanoku. She leads the National Youth Orchestra, and she's a famous double bassist who was a pupil at Blean school in the 1960s. Chi Chi emailed Jenny, my deputy, during the latter stages of my secondment, to see if she could come into school to use the hall, and to use the children to help her with producing a video to go with her latest CD. Well, this is quite an honour for the school, and we're delighted to be able to help. Chi Chi came in today and did some filming with us, and was superb. Clearly she is a gifted musician and a bubbly personality. After the recording, we had time to chat in my office, and got out the school log books. She enjoyed reminiscing about herself and her brother, who also attended the school, and we found them listed in the admissions register. Also, interestingly enough, her brother was in the punishment book for some relatively minor misdemeanour! She was delighted about this little record which was unknown to her. I made copies of the relevant entries for her to take away to share with her family.

She also was a very able and competent sprinter, in fact she almost got to international level before a knee injury halted that career and gave her the impetus to focus on music. As it was a lovely sunny day she was very keen to go out on the field at break time as the running track was already marked out for the summer term. Chi Chi the eminent musician was revisiting her childhood on our field by racing against 11-year-old girls and boys, and really enjoying that, before coming back to my office really fired up about winning certain races – all good fun.

4th May – Canterbury

Today I attended another session of the M.Ed. course. I'm now finding it quite hard. Re-establishing myself at school and doing the M.Ed. is proving quite difficult. Lately it has been a challenge to find the time, the energy and the concentration to be able to manage combining the two, and this is surprising me because I normally enjoy work and study and can usually take them in my stride.

5th May – Margate

Today began normally. The sun was shining. The *BBC Breakfast* weather girl predicted warm sunshine, which pleased me as a trip in the sun is always better than in the rain. I had dinner duty awaiting me at school, and it is much less hassle if the children are able to run around outside. Because it's so dry and warm they would have the added bonus of going on the field to play.

We arrived at Queen Elizabeth The Queen Mother Hospital for my rearranged appointment with the neurologist a little early because I hate being late and were shown into the waiting area by a friendly receptionist. I remember glancing at my watch and the time was 10.15. My mind drifted to what would be happening at school; it would be assembly now and the theme was one about being positive, with the hymn 'One More Step Along the World I Go'.

Exactly on time the neurologist's nurse called me in to have my weight and blood pressure checked. All routine. I was led back into the waiting room. Break time back at school now, again thank goodness for the sunshine.

Thoughts of school were interrupted by 'Mr Oliver, will you please come this way.' Rosemary and I were led across the waiting area to a typical doctor's consultation room. Square. Modern. Paperwork strewn across a table. Computer screen idling on the corner of a desk. NHS files much like the Department for Education equivalents in my office. And there centre stage was the neurologist who until this moment had been merely a name on an appointment letter. In the next few moments this was to change.

The consultant invited us to take a seat and posed a series of questions about my health, and why I had gone to my GP a month or so previously. I explained about the falls, the tiredness and my inability to concentrate. He listened intently before embarking on a series of what I regarded as silly questions – what month is it, what season, who is the prime minister, count back from 70 in 7s – all very easy. Then onto him reading three words and asking me to repeat them – I hadn't a clue. Where are we at this moment – I couldn't remember the name of the hospital but knew it's in Margate, wasn't that good enough? Then the three words/objects again – still they didn't register. He paused and turned our attention to his computer screen. I felt at this moment like I was having an out-of-body experience – as if I wasn't present in the room.

He broke the silence with...

'Well Mr Oliver, I think that the results of your scan and what you have said to me today is consistent with early stages of Alzheimer's disease.'

He went on to explain that the GP had referred me for the scan to rule out a brain tumour. He assured me there was no tumour. Along with Alzheimer's, this was the first time this had been mentioned.

I was speechless. My wife was speechless. The consultant sensed this, and went on to explain that this was a suggested diagnosis and lots more tests and scans would be required in order for this to be confirmed. He then drew two helpful pictures, showing, as he described it, a healthy 54-year-old brain; and then he drew mine based on the scan – he did try to explain the scan to us but it was too difficult to draw sense from it. The comparisons the drawings illustrated were helpful. By now I was regaining some sense of the moment, and the dialogue I felt was necessary. The first question revolved around the subsequent tests and scans, then we moved to talk about carrying on working, which I wanted to do.

Next we raised the question of our forthcoming, long-booked, annual trip to Australia. We were alarmed by his response to this which was...not to go. But everything was planned and paid for. His advice remained the same.

The sun was still shining as we emerged from the confines of the hospital. I suggested to Rosemary, 'Let's have a walk on the beach nearby' – a favourite spot of ours, to clear our heads and take stock – 'and I'll ring school to get someone to cover my lunch duty.' That's what we did, and I turned to Rosemary the moment we felt the sand under our feet, and I said, 'One door closes and one door will open.' I didn't know which door it would be.

I arrived back at school at around 2.30 p.m., and Rosemary and I met with the three secretaries and the three senior teaching staff. I'd phoned the secretary earlier to arrange a meeting with them, and they were all able to get out of class and to leave the children with a teaching assistant for a few minutes whilst they heard what I wanted to explain to them. I went through the morning with them, and they were immensely shocked. I drew for them the same sketch that the neurologist had drawn for us to show a healthy 54-year-old brain, and mine, with the word 'atrophy' clearly written next to the spaces between my skull and my brain. Once the shock started to subside for them I led us to talk about plans for the future.

I have decided to tell a small, trusted group of senior staff as I felt it was too much responsibility for one person alone. Now they can confide in each other and hopefully watch out for me and help me through this potentially difficult time as I want to carry on working for as long as is possible. Nothing as yet is confirmed – we told them this four or five times in this short meeting. We began to set in place a strategy which would allow me to carry on working for as long as possible. I wrote out the plan with them which I pinned on my office notice board behind some timetables – only they and I knew this was there. I asked Ginny, my secretary, to cancel a meeting set for 2.30 with the special educational needs governor, who I will now meet later in the week.

When I got home from work I rang the GP to tell him about my appointment, and whilst trying to make some sense of what the day had brought I told him something about what had been said to me by the neurologist. The coin dropped – this links back to the conversation that he and I had, a week or so ago, when he said to listen carefully to the neurologist. My GP attentively heard my account and to me he seemed very surprised, because he said that Alzheimer's was not on his radar. I don't think he had met someone of my age and in my position with dementia before, although all of us reminded ourselves that this is only a suggested diagnosis, and is not confirmed, so we are hopeful that the neurologist has got it wrong at this stage.

6th May – Blean

Not much time to come to terms with yesterday's substantial happenings and messages. I've just had to try and absorb it and get on with what I'm doing at the moment. So today, I've got a PTFA (Parents, Teachers and Friends Association) meeting, and a head teacher area meeting.

7th May – Canterbury

At the heads' meeting there was a lot of conversation about me returning back to the fold, and leaving the other side of the fence, along with a lot of good banter, but you can imagine what was at the back of my mind.

Obviously, no one else would know – I'm not telling anyone else at this stage because there is no need to do so yet and it would make my professional position far more difficult.

8th May – Canterbury

When I saw the neurologist two days ago he gave me a form to have some blood tests done, so this morning I went off to Kent and Canterbury Hospital with Rosemary, and had some blood samples taken for thyroid, diabetes, vitamin B, plus some other things that I can't remember. I guess, from what he said to me, this was to rule out other possible explanations for my symptoms. After this it was back to school, and a normal day if there is now such a thing.

10th May – Blean

I had my first telephone conversation today with Kim, who is the neurologist's secretary at Margate Hospital. She was really helpful, and very understanding, and is willing to be a port of call if I have things I want to ask, or things I want to check and to know more about. You cannot imagine the relief I felt when she said, 'You must ring me, it's not a problem, here's my number in the office, and these are the hours I work.' That's the first medical prop that I have felt, alongside the GP, Rosemary and the senior staff at school. After this call I then had some meetings at the school, with both Hilary, my SENCO (special educational needs coordinator), who is doing a fantastic job with the special needs children in the school, and Pam, the bursar, to go through the school finances for the year end, and planning for next year's finances. I always find this exercise exciting as we seek to make the school even more efficient for everyone – children, staff and parents.

12th May – Blean

Today was a governor's meeting, the first one since my return to school. Governors don't know anything about the neurologist appointment and what transpired from that. It was a very straightforward meeting and everything, as far as they're concerned, seems in order for the school and my return to it. I am finding it hard though, dealing with the diagnosis, and clearly my health isn't as I'd wish it to be, which is such a shame as I was so looking forward to coming back to school. I'm still enjoying the job, but finding that my health is giving more concern than I would wish it to, and I need to think more about how I can manage this.

13th May – Canterbury

One thing to help me with my health, I've decided, is to return to the Ideal Spine Centre, which I left a couple of years ago. Rosemary has been a paying patient there since soon after it opened. I spent one year there, and then left, and now it appears as though returning, and having weekly chiropractic care, alongside a fortnightly deep tissue massage, is going to help me. There are other things that the centre provides, such as talks and advice around holistic healthcare. I went to see Christian who runs the centre today and restarted. I hope this is going to be helpful in maintaining my health.

14th May – Blean

High on my list of priorities is staff contracts, as many members of staff were on temporary contracts during the course of my secondment. With the support of the senior leadership team, I've been working hard in trying to manage and consider how we're going to address this, and which key members of staff we can look to put onto substantive permanent contracts. One of the teachers, who is on a temporary contract, has been becoming quite agitated by the fact that perhaps I haven't been giving it the speediest of attention that she would wish, due to a number of considerations, not the least of which being my health, and today she came to see me. We had a really productive conversation, at the end of which I gave her a consoling hug which surprised me, because I don't remember ever doing that before with a colleague. Not a big issue, but alongside the conversation it seemed to help in that situation, and it showed her that I do care, and that I do want to try and resolve this to the satisfaction of her and the school.

18th May – Canterbury

Having given more thought since the last master's course session on 4th May, I went today to see the director of the course to explain that because of my diagnosis, and my health, I no longer feel able to continue with the master's. I can't see what support they or anyone else can give me. I sense that the decline is beginning, and I've just got to manage this as best as I possibly can. Upon hearing my diagnosis Robin's unsurprising response was,

'Well, we'd better call it a day then.' Understandably, there was no offer of support, there was no offer of encouragement, or desire to persuade me to change my mind, so that appears to be it. This is a real shame, because the course was going well; my marks were between 62 and 73 per cent, which were in line for a very good master's qualification; plus though hard, I was really enjoying the stimulation of the course. But it's not to be, I've got to cut my losses a bit I guess, and focus on what is important.

21st May – Canterbury

I attended a neurophysiology EEG (electroencephalogram) scan at Kent and Canterbury Hospital, the results of which will be shared with the neurologist and me at my next appointment with him. Later the education welfare officer came in to see me, just to touch base about the attendance of the pupils at school, which is, generally speaking, good. I suspect it was as much a courtesy call as anything. Later in the day I had a meeting at another local school, with a colleague, and then headed off to Nottingham with Rosemary to visit my parents for the weekend.

3rd June – Canterbury

I saw the GP about the appointment with the neurologist, and went through the updates that have occurred since last time I saw him. He checked how I was getting on at work and how I was feeling, and then tested my blood pressure. It was useful to have a conversation with him.

On the way out of the GP's I popped into the chemist next door, and spent £4.95 on a copy of a really useful book by Nori Graham and James Warner, called *Understanding Alzheimer's Disease and Other Dementias*. I think it will be supportive as I go through this process, because it takes the reader through all the complex tests and explains the different dementias. I realise I know very little about dementia other than the fact that five weeks ago I would have believed it to be an old person's disease; I never realised it could possibly affect someone of my age, least of all me.

6th June – Whitstable

For a week or two now, Rosemary's been picking me up from school at lunchtime, once, twice or sometimes three times a week, to go out around midday when I'm not doing lunch duties and have no lunchtime meetings planned. This gives me a break from school and a rest. Today we went to Seasalter and sat by the beach in the car, with a sandwich followed by a snooze, before returning to school for the afternoon.

On other occasions, when I've had less time available to me, we've just gone to the car park in Blean Woods and done the same, which has proved just as restful and restorative.

10th June – Blean

As I recorded in my diary a few weeks ago, there's been lots of interviews required for moving staff from temporary contracts to permanent contracts. Today was a bit different, in the sense that I was interviewing for a new reception class teacher, and we appointed someone new to the staff to fill a vacancy.

I do enjoy interviewing, although at the moment there's just too many of them to be done to enjoy it, but it needs to be done, and it is satisfying when you get a successful outcome at the end. I am fortunate to be able to share the role with my deputies Jenny and Rachael, alongside a supportive governor.

18th June – Blean

Open evening. There was a very good atmosphere at the school; lots of parents attended, and lots of positive comments were expressed by people coming up to me and saying they were pleased to see me back in school, all of which was gratifying to hear and reinforced my positive thought about leaving the advisor role to return to the fold.

I had a successful day today, where I felt good. I had a break at lunchtime, again with Rosemary, so that helped to sustain me for the long day and evening in school.

21st June – Blean

We had a visitor come to the school to do a drumming workshop with the children. He was the drummer from Status Quo, and to record the event we had Neil Bell, who is the parent of two boys in the school, and works for the BBC as a local sports reporter. Today he reverted to his cameraman role, and brought equipment to record the event for the BBC. I look forward to watching it tonight on the local news.

22nd June – Whitstable

An appointment with the local education authority, to discuss issues around occupational health, and either sustaining me in the job (with support) or looking for an exit strategy and potential retirement. I want to keep as many options open as I can, so that when any decisions need to be made, I'm in the best place possible to make them. So today's meeting, with the local authority represented by Annette Kelly, was really helpful because as always she gave me good advice from Human Resources (HR) which should hopefully help me steer my way through the next few months in deciding what is best for myself, and what is best for the school.

23rd June – Canterbury

After reflecting upon the neurologist's advice to cancel our trip to Australia set for August, we have confirmed in our mind that we *will* still go, and although we have changed the itinerary slightly we are determined to go. I wrote to him on 8th June and explained this alongside more information about our previous positive experience of long-distance travel and the fact that the holiday will in part be with Aussie friends made during our year living there in 1989. In fairness, a letter arrived from him today to say that his recommendation not to travel was based upon the scan and tests, and if I felt well enough he would leave it to me to decide on this. I am left with the thought that it would have been easy to have taken his advice at a point when we felt immensely vulnerable, and therefore not to embark upon our trip to Australia and beyond that never to go again. Time will tell if we have still got more trips left in us.

30th June – Blean

I spent the last couple of days reading through 460 school reports. Most of them were very good. It's an incredibly difficult task because they are about three or four pages long, and by the time I get to the end of a report, I have to re-read certain sections before I make a comment because I cannot remember now what I've read. It is terribly frustrating because I've done this for a number of years without this problem. The reading and retaining, and then acting upon, is becoming much, much more difficult and frustrating. I want to get it right, and also, I have a duty, which I place upon myself, of checking the reports to be 100 per cent accurate. Most are good, but there are one or two teachers who require me to make quite a few corrections. I don't want anything going home to parents that is not correct.

9th July – Blean

The weather today wasn't great, which was a shame, and so our school's summer fair was slightly impeded by that. It wasn't a lovely summer evening, but it was largely dry and most of the events were able to take place outside. Again, a very good turnout by parents, children and staff, and after counting up at the end of the day, it looks like we've gone well past £4000 again. Last year, it was closer to £5000, but then it was a beautifully warm summer evening. Hopefully all the parents and staff who worked so hard on the event will be pleased with the result.

14th July – Margate

I saw the neurologist again today for the second consultation with him, having not seen him since the original bomb shell was dropped in May, although Kim has been very understanding and supportive on the phone if I've needed any advice. I have re-read and tried to make sense of his report a number of times, along with the letters he has written and copied me into to my GP. Phrases like 'high-functioning individual with memory problems', 'I am concerned that this gentleman has early Alzheimer's disease', 'moderate to marked parietal atrophy on the MRI scan' and 'delayed recall' jumped off the page. Today, he discharged me from the hospital, and is going to start the ball rolling in regard to appointments at the memory clinic. His use of the word 'discharged' worried me greatly as it will mean another step into the unknown, and now without the considerate support of his secretary. He gave me some more tests, and seems more convinced than ever that it is Alzheimer's. I'm still not sure, I really don't know what it is I'm contending with, but I do know that I need to go through this process in order to get answers to these questions.

Alongside these extra tests, he gave me the results of the blood tests, all of which he said have come back as satisfactory, which in some ways is good. However, the hope we had was that maybe something less significant would be shown within those blood tests, meaning it wasn't Alzheimer's. It appears that the options are narrowing down to just one or two, and Alzheimer's, he says, is the most likely. So I'll await an appointment from the memory clinic, and obviously respond to that and attend and hopefully show what I can still do successfully.

Having seen the professor in the morning, in the afternoon it was a lighter time for me because a samba band came into school and did a workshop with the children. I was able to sit in for a few minutes and it's lovely to see them enjoying something like that, and to take my mind off what's been happening elsewhere in my life. After school, the reports went home, and our staff meeting which followed began with a sigh of relief! Now the focus is on bringing the school to a close for the end of term.

At the staff meeting I told the staff about my health concerns, and in the evening raised the same with the governors; before going in I did so privately with Hugh, the chairman of the governors. But I didn't tell them what I was dealing with because I don't know at this stage. I just said that it wasn't contagious and I am not in the best of health (which I think they had twigged anyway; they had already begun to realise that things weren't right with my health). Staff were very quiet, and I could see that people were thinking deeply about what I was saying to them, and you can't say more than that. People have been very supportive since I've been back to school, but have also been quite anxious about not knowing what it is that is different with the boss. For example, I have had conversations with John the caretaker around me not remembering the code for the alarm to the school, which was previously not a problem. I don't know what he thinks of that. Also, whereas before my office door was always open, now there are periods in the day when it has to be closed as I cannot focus on doing my job with my door open because of the distractions that sometimes brings. Previously I'd easily ignored them.

So I thought it was useful at this stage, particularly with the summer holiday approaching, to tell staff that there are concerns, but that it's not catching, it's not going to kill me off in the short term, and just to try and put people's minds at ease, whilst making them aware that I am struggling a little with my health.

15th July – Canterbury

With Rosemary's support I had my first appointment arranged by HR at the local authority, with occupational health. It really was just a check-up in order to make them aware of what I'm dealing with, by way of a suspected diagnosis (no more than that), and what I am putting in place at work to enable me to carry on, and to enable other people and myself to remain safe and secure in the work environment. I was mindful of what the neurologist said to me when I last saw him and mentioned this appointment today. He said, 'If you show them my report they will finish you tomorrow.' These words were ringing in my mind, so I withheld his report; if and when I do have to end working I want it to be at the right time for me.

I approached it as a straightforward appointment. It took place at the University of Kent health centre. I was told I would get a report in due course; I hope it'll say, this guy is okay to carry on working because of what he's putting in place at the moment.

16th July – Canterbury and Nottingham

I missed the governors meeting tonight because Rosemary rang me to say that my dad had a heart attack today. There had been a phone call to her from the hospital, and he's been admitted to Nottingham Hospital. So tonight, after I've done my diary and finished at work, we'll head off to Nottingham for the weekend, and see how things are. I've told the governors that unfortunately I've got to miss the meeting and have explained why.

23rd July – School breaks up

End of term and as always each day I said goodbye to the children and parents at the gate and expressed my hope that they all have a wonderful break. Next was a walk around to the classrooms to say the same to the staff. I look forward to seeing them all again, refreshed, in September, and I look forward to that for myself.

28th July–27th August – Sydney, Darwin, the Ghan railway, Alice Springs, Adelaide

The trip that nearly didn't happen! All went brilliantly well. We flew easily into Sydney where we were able to enjoy an extended stay with our dear friend Sue who having recently lost her husband was pleased to have our company for longer than originally planned. To make the trip more manageable and in the light of the neurologist's advice, we skipped the Cairns element of the original plan and next headed straight up to the tropics for a few hot and sultry days in Darwin. Last time there, in 1994, we went in the footsteps of Crocodile Dundee and were rather more adventurous; this time gentle strolls were more the order of the day. Darwin also gave us the starting point for a much-anticipated trip on the iconic Ghan train heading south through the centre of Australia. The trip truly lived up to our expectations and was luxury on the rails – our own cabin with room service and shower, superb dining and great Aussie company from strangers keen to share yarns and life stories. We broke the journey in Alice Springs which again was a revisit, this time previously seen in 1989 during the year we spent in the country whilst I was on a teacher exchange. Alice is an amazing place – hundreds of miles from anywhere and surrounded by bush and desert which extended right up to the rear of our hotel and which we sat admiring as the sun went down over the MacDonnell Ranges each day. We also ventured out of town by minibus to experience walking amongst the prehistoric cycads adorning Palm Valley. Saying goodbye in the Ghan to Alice Springs was hard, but the enticement of Adelaide was a strong magnet. We spent another 24 hours in the luxury of the train before disembarking into the arms of friends Alan and Glenys in Adelaide, in whose company we had a fabulous couple of weeks.

Will there be another trip to our beloved Australia? Never say never. A lesson maybe to those medical experts who write off those of us with dementia all too easily at times.

31st August – Blean

Last day of the school holiday. I returned to work after the summer break and the trip to Australia. I began by feeling refreshed and ready to start the term, but also, there are some days which I would liken life to being in a fog that descends. It's an unusual feeling. I've never had it before, but the last few months had some 'foggy days'. However, most days for me are pretty sunny and quite clear. But there are some days when, really, I don't function at all well. Today developed into one of those. It became a foggy day. I returned to work and pottered about feeling as if I was on a ship in rough seas and then had another fall, followed at the end of work with a finance meeting which I have little recall of.

1st September – Blean

The sun was shining inside and out today. I led staff training in the morning around looking forward to a new term, with time constructively spent planning in year groups and confirming dates as a whole staff for the term ahead. After the talk I gave back in July to staff about my health, I suspect one or two people thought I wouldn't be there, but everyone seemed very pleased that I was. We had a productive day, and in the afternoon I was able to work quietly in my office, and prepare for the new school year.

3rd September – Blean

Two outwardly good days in school, but deep down quite traumatic for me, because I do have a sense that things are slipping, and I'm not that sure how much longer I am going to be able to sustain myself in work. I decided to go and see the GP tonight, so I rang him this afternoon, and booked an appointment after school.

4th September – Canterbury

I did go to the GP yesterday, and not surprisingly, he said, 'Really, you cannot continue like this. You cannot continue doing what you are doing at work with all that's happening to your health, so I'm going to sign you off.' He took the decision away from me, and said, 'I'm going to sign you off for two months, which will be an initial period, and during that time, I think you've really got to sit down and think seriously about your future, Keith, and about maybe starting the ball rolling regarding early retirement.' This is the first time I've had that level of conversation, either with him or with anybody, so it was quite a sobering experience to confront the reality of my situation. But I sensed it was coming, and it was no great surprise really, so I'll see how we go in the next two months, take the time off, take stock, and give myself time and space to see what the future holds. I am not scared of what this all means but I am confused, and 1001 thoughts whizz around in my mind – retire/work, retire/work...dementia...Alzheimer's...end.

6th September – Canterbury

First day of sick leave. Last Saturday, 4th September, without people knowing what I'm contending with, Rosemary and I went to Flatford Mill with the Canterbury Arts Society for a day trip. John, my school caretaker, was there, with his partner Jean. I didn't say anything about my health. Rosemary and I were determined if possible to have a good day with them and the rest of the group, because Flatford has always been a very special place to me, having taken children there for many years on residential visits, and also taken staff from both Blean and Barton on day trips there. Rosemary and I took our son James a few years ago so he could have a look. It's a wonderful place, with the John Constable associations, and the positive memories that it has for me as a teacher leading residential visits there with children between 1992 and 2005.

Interestingly enough, last night on the weather forecast, it was saying there was a stormy spell of weather about to happen. I said to Rosemary, 'It's lucky we're not venturing far tomorrow, because of the storms.' She said, 'I wish you hadn't told me that.' And my response to that was, 'Well, I'm not too worried Rosemary, because I won't remember tomorrow what I've said.' Hopefully we can retain our sense of humour.

9th September – Canterbury

There was a piece in the *Kentish Gazette* villages section for Blean where Godfrey, the village correspondent, had picked up on a newsletter I'd written to parents to inform them that I was going to need to take some time off due to my health concerns, and that Lynne Lawrence would stand in as the acting head during my period of absence.

18th September – Canterbury

At one time the thought of retirement had some appeal, but not in these circumstances. I had always envisaged myself travelling or gardening either independently or with Rosemary. Spending days watching daytime TV is really *so* boring, and when I summon enthusiasm to watch a film I have to make notes in an exercise book as to what the film is called and what it was about because otherwise I have no recall of watching it.

21st September – Canterbury

Having travelled many times past St Martin's Hospital on the outskirts of Canterbury, today is the first time that I have crossed its threshold. Whilst the grounds are green and pleasant the building is quite foreboding, and was a raw reminder of many hours painfully spent visiting my mother in similar institutions in Nottingham. Consequently, I felt anxious attending my first appointment today at the memory clinic, where I saw a consultant named Dr Aston, and a nurse. The process seemed well organised and they put me through some brief cognitive assessments, one of which seemed vaguely familiar and reminded me of the 20 questions the neurologist had asked me, especially the three words I was asked to remember – again I could not recall them; I also had some physical health checks, and a reading test – something I have delivered for the past 33 years but not done myself for over 40 years. I think there were more tests but didn't note them down; otherwise all I recall is that most of the questions seemed very easy, apart from when they 'tricked' me and asked me to remember what they had just told me.

Also today, I finished reading *My Bonnie*, a book by John Suchet about his wife who had young onset dementia. I've decided to start to read more about dementia, because if that is what I'm contending with, I want to know more about it so that I'm better prepared, and better able to deal with what it throws at me. Rosemary does not want to read it. My response is that knowledge is power and I really want to try and exert some kind of control over what I'm living with at the moment. Reading *My Bonnie* didn't help me a lot. It was a love story by a husband/carer, and it was a very sad love story, but it was interesting to read the point of view of somebody who had actually lived through something that, if this diagnosis is confirmed, Rosemary and I may well live through in the future.

25th September – Nottingham

A traumatic day as my dad, who's been very, very ill recently after his heart attack in the summer, died this morning. He died at 9.30, and we heard the news in the car on the A1 near Peterborough whilst on route to Nottingham to see him. The hospital rang me at 9.50 on my mobile to say he had died. We arrived at the hospital just before 1 p.m., and stayed with him until about 2.15. He simply looked asleep. We saw Jane, my cousin, and Maisie, my aunt, who had been with him. Whilst feeling very sad I also felt a sense of release for Dad, because at 82 he had been reasonably well until the last three or four months during which he had gone downhill quite rapidly. The heart attack and the stomach cancer had really taken their toll recently. He didn't want to have any kind of chemotherapy, or any other treatment, so really he was prepared and willing to pass on, and thankfully he didn't have to suffer for long.

So now to make the arrangements for the funeral, and everything else that's required. We plan to spend some time in Nottingham using his council bungalow as a base, and then moving between Canterbury and

Nottingham whilst I plan and address what needs to be done to settle his affairs. I hope that I am up to the task.

4th October – Nottingham

Today was Dad's funeral at Wilford Crematorium and there was a pleasing turnout from friends and family. Whilst it was warming to see family who I had not seen for many years brought together by the occasion, it was sad that it took a funeral to achieve this. My mother was brought along by the care home staff. It was traumatic and distressing for her, and for everyone else, because she found it terribly hard, and called out constantly during the service despite our efforts to console and pacify her.

Then afterwards, those of us who were able to went for a meal at a pub in Bunny nearby. I chose this partly for its convenient location, and also because it was the last pub we took my dad to a few months previously.

16th October – Canterbury

I've been in contact with Lynne, the acting head at school who's covering my absence, and we agreed about reducing my visits to the school, and that I should focus on trying to get well. I am confident she will manage the school very efficiently. She did add that I'm welcome to call in if I wish to see colleagues socially. I'm not sure whether I will or not. Time will tell. But at this stage, I think my priority is on focusing on the health assessments, and trying to adjust to life away from school, thus giving each of us the space to do what we need to do.

18th October – Blean

I did go into school today with Lynne's agreement, to update staff, because it's now been six weeks since I've been off sick, and clearly they're wondering how I am and what it is I'm dealing with. I spoke to the teachers, the teaching assistants and John the caretaker as one group, really just to tell them where we're at, and to bring them up to speed with the confidential and unconfirmed diagnosis that I have got young onset dementia, which is Alzheimer's in my case. I did stress to them that it's not been confirmed yet, but it is looking more and more likely, and consequently, almost certain that I will not be returning to school. As I read what I had prepared I did look up many times into the 40 or more faces in front of me and you could have heard a pin drop. Never have I seen a group of people in the collective, stunned hush that blanketed the classroom we were in. I could not speak afterwards and left silently.

19th October – Canterbury

The last two entries in my journal and diary were difficult to write. I had said that one door closes and one door opens – I can sense the closing but as yet there is no opening door in sight.

Today I went to Kent and Canterbury Hospital for the next round of investigations, this time for a SPECT (single photon emission computerised tomography) brain scan (also known as an HMPAO (hexamethylpropyleneamine oxime) scan). With the knowledge taken from my treasured Graham and Warner book, I recognised this as where they put a sort of hair net on me and I see all sorts of brightly coloured images on the screen. From this they can tell how messages are being transferred around the brain, although for me it simply reminded me of a psychedelic album cover from the late 60s. I didn't really understand it. It wasn't painful, it wasn't uncomfortable, and as I left I was thinking that it would be another piece in the jigsaw and that the picture must be emerging for the professionals to help me.

22nd October – Canterbury

I went to see the GP for updates on how things were going. I told him about the first appointment at the memory clinic, and he really simply used the appointment as an opportunity to reinforce his earlier conversation with me about my need to consider retirement. I don't know what to do. On the one hand I'm still not keen to retire because I don't know what it is I'm dealing with, and I really want to get more appointments under my belt, so that I know for certain what it is that I'm confronting; on the other hand all I read about Alzheimer's shows me that if it is confirmed I cannot carry on working.

3rd November – Canterbury

Today it was back to St Martin's for the first assessment at the memory clinic with a clinical psychologist named Dr Elizabeth Field, and her assistant psychologist Jouko Koecher. It seemed quite straightforward – lots of questions, both written and spoken, and at the end I just came out feeling very tired. I was able to tell Dr Field how I was, and what it was I was dealing with, and as a result I hope she got to know me a little as a person.

10th November – Canterbury

Second assessment appointment at the memory clinic, with the same two people: Dr Field and Jouko. Pretty much like the first one really, although a bit less talking this time, and more written tests.

16th November – Canterbury

Third assessment appointment, again with the same two people, Dr Field and Jouko. I took lots of notes with me explaining how I felt. Now I know and trust them more, I feel better able to confide in them what I'm dealing with, and feel that my assessment is progressing satisfactorily. At each appointment they are giving me feedback on the results, and they range from being average to being well below average. In fact, for one set of assessments, they told me I was in the bottom fifth percentile, which was very alarming. That was an assessment where they read me a story, and then asked me questions on it, a bit like a comprehension exercise. Normally this would be very easy, but I found it incredibly difficult because I couldn't remember what they'd said to me. I said, 'It's a bit like those ball bearings and that physics motion where one ball bearing knocks out another ball bearing, or two ball bearings knock two ball bearings out. Is this called a Newton's Cradle?' As I tried to cling onto what information I was being told, the new piece of information was knocking the old piece out of my brain. I had not been referred to as average since my secondary school days in French – which I hated and thought I was rubbish at – and as for being in the bottom 5 per cent of anything cognitive, that is a totally new and alien feeling.

All this was immensely disconcerting and caused me a lot of psychological problems. I was trying so hard. Going into these tests, I really wanted to score as high as I could, so that they would tell me at the end of the day it wasn't Alzheimer's but maybe it was something else.

20th November – Canterbury

Feeling physically okay, but very tired, and when we spoke to Jouko about this on 16th November, he came up with a really good answer, which was that the brain is a very hungry organ, and is causing this tiredness, because I'm having to work much harder to remain in the same place, and to do things that, previously, I didn't have to work as hard at doing. This gives me a sense of frustration and, I guess, another reason why something like a fog begins to descend. Whether the frustration is causing the fog or whether the fog causes the frustration, I'm not sure, but the two seem very entwined with each other.

I'm also having trouble remembering and following what I watch on television. Because the weather now is not very good, I'm not able to enjoy days in the garden. I am less able to do physical things to keep me well and keep me occupied, and I'm watching more television, which leaves me bored, and frustrated that I cannot follow or remember the programmes and films. I continue to keep an exercise book, where I write in something about the film, and then test myself. I watch the film, and then I try to write a summary of the film, to challenge myself on what I can remember.

Also, Tom, one of the teachers at Blean, very kindly visited me the other day and brought me the complete catalogue of *Steptoe and Son* as a boxed set on DVD. I've started to watch them and I'm quite enjoying reconnecting to my youth. Also, the episodes are quite short (about 25 minutes) and I can just about retain my concentration for that time, but there is a limit to the number of Steptoes you can watch in a day, however much I like them!

30th November – Canterbury

I was due to have a final appointment today at the memory clinic, but there's been an unusually high snowfall overnight and this morning, which has meant that the appointment has had to be cancelled as staff cannot get into the clinic, but the caller reassured me that it will be rescheduled.

6th December – Canterbury

Thankfully I have not had to wait long and the snow soon cleared, allowing me to attend the fourth and final appointment at the memory clinic to get the results of the last batch of tests and to hear the summary and conclusions from Dr Field and Jouko. They didn't confirm the diagnosis of dementia, but told me that I'll have another appointment soon with Dr Aston, the psychiatrist who I met a few months ago at the first appointment at the memory clinic. I don't remember seeing her since. It is her role to tell me what the results mean. Having said that, both Dr Field and Jouko are mindful that it is looking very much like she will say it is Alzheimer's.

7th December – Canterbury

Dr Field's words are ringing in my ears today. I keep asking myself how I feel about this. Having so often used the word 'unconfirmed' over the past seven months, it is now being removed from my vocabulary. On the other hand, part of me is relieved that now we know what it is we are dealing with and can hopefully, with support, move forward and consider the future, albeit a future which was never in our plans.

21st December – Canterbury

We had the initial visit from Sinead McGettrick, the Admiral Nurse, who came to see us both at home. Admiral Nurses, who are specialist dementia nurses, are an invaluable support, mainly for carers, but also possibly for people with a diagnosis, and Sinead came over as both a very nice person and a very able practitioner, who I hope and expect will be a great ally to us in the future.

She visited us at home, and checked how we were. I also think there was an element of her seeing what the home environment is like, how we responded to each other, and how we responded to her. It all seemed very straightforward and very positive, and actually quite constructive and helpful.

31st December – Canterbury Memory Clinic

I certainly won't be going out celebrating tonight, though it is not as if New Year's Eve has ever been a great cause for celebration for Rosemary and me. We have usually seen the new year in, but we've not been ones for partying necessarily, although there have been a few over the years. But not tonight, because today was an important appointment for us at the memory clinic to see Dr Aston, supported by Jouko. Having Jouko there was very helpful as he is a more familiar face to me than Dr Aston and I felt more at ease. During the four assessments I got a sense that we were building up to this moment. I suspected there would be few surprises in what I was told and that any surprises, positive or not, would arise from the way Rosemary and I took the information I was about to hear. Dr Aston explained, very compassionately, the reports and the assessments that Dr

Field and Jouko have done over the past few months and how they built upon the neurologist's reports. She then explained to me that they were all very suggestive of a diagnosis of Alzheimer's with a possibility that there's an element of vascular dementia in there as well. She followed this with the assurance that I will be getting some after-diagnosis support, but she wasn't sure what it would be, and that she would keep me on her books as the person responsible for managing my care alongside my GP, and that I would see her for an appointment at some point in the new year.

So, with this relatively short appointment, I now have the diagnosis but hopefully not the label 'demented'.

So, dear diary, looking into the new year, we'll see what 2011 brings.

Sometime in 2010

Dear Alzheimer's

I realised that you have been watching me for some time, sitting on my shoulder as my mother developed Alzheimer's and you strove to rob us of her personality and her love. You failed with both, because even though eventually she did pass away you didn't take her.

Having returned to school today from seeing the neurologist I recognised your presence within the room. I am not going to say there is anything positive about meeting you because there isn't, and I hope our association is one which I can handle. I also recognise those early symptoms which I was able to dismiss, and I respect your tenacity in not giving up in your efforts to get the better of me. The neurologist's words about Rosemary and me cancelling Australia were I know fed to him by you. I hope you recognise my defiance in saying to both him and you, 'We are going. Bugger you Dementia!' I suspect that you may accompany us on our trip. I hope not, and I will certainly do my very best to leave you behind.

Why don't you come out of the misty shadows where you lurk? Why don't you have the courage to talk with me about why it is that on the days you seek to spoil my life I sway, wobble and struggle to concentrate, like I've been on the biggest booze cruise imaginable without the thirst-quenching pleasure or the delight of reaching a comfortable safe harbour? There again, the hangover that *you* deliver won't last, and the sun, after a boozy hangover compounds the strife with you, brings relief, and always will do so.

I know these are the earliest of days in our relationship and I hope to win more exchanges than I lose with you over the coming years.

Your far from obedient servant

Keith

2011

—

'Establishing a new life'

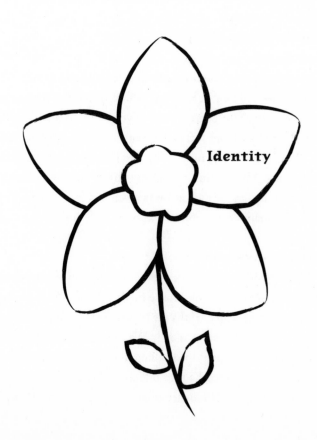

Identity

4th January – Canterbury

I have been thinking a lot about my visit today to the GP for the results of my latest assessment and to discuss early retirement with him, an option which seems ever more likely. He gave me a prescription for a medication called escitalopram (5 mg). He told me to increase it in two weeks' time to 10 mg by taking two tablets. I wasn't very happy about this, so I said I would take the prescription on the understanding that I no longer had to take the Keppra, which the neurologist started me on back in May, just in case I was suffering from epilepsy. This was because of my very poor concentration and petit mal-type symptoms. I didn't think I had any epilepsy, but that's what he gave me as a precaution.

I disputed with the GP the need for the antidepressants because I don't feel depressed. What I was looking for, really, was anti-Alzheimer's disease drugs, but that wasn't forthcoming. To keep him appeased I agreed to that prescription, although I am unsure if I will collect the tablets.

5th January – Canterbury

Once a month, during the winter, we meet as a small U3A (University of the Third Age) group at one of our houses to discuss family history. My focus in the past has been to look at Rosemary's family, and I've tracked back her maternal side to the 18th century. Now I've got some time on my hands, allied with the ancestry.com software given to me as part of my retirement gift from Blean, I can devote time to my family as my knowledge ends with my grandparents. My last link to a grandparent was my mother's dad, a policeman, who died in 1963 when I was seven; my father's dad, who was a coal miner, died many years before I was born.

11th January – Whitstable

I had a meeting with a local education authority officer, Annette, about my retirement process at Brook House in Whitstable. With her help and Rosemary's support I completed the retirement forms, and they've now been sent off to the Teacher Pension Agency. We concentrated on my difficulties around cognitive functioning; form filling, for example, has become much more difficult and I do need help to understand and then complete them. Having Annette alongside Rosemary and me was a great help. When leaving the office Rosemary and I could not get over the fact that the chairs were screwed to the floor – this was a social services office and we were told the concern was they could be used as a weapon against officers!

17th January – Whitstable

I am trying to establish a routine, and on Tuesday mornings Rosemary goes to an art lesson in Whitstable, which gives me an opportunity to go for a walk along the beach. Irrespective of the weather I do enjoy this. In fact, winter days like today which are crisp and bright after an early frost are invigorating. It's very quiet. I factor in an hour during this walk to go into the library to use their computer system, because I can access more websites for family history, alongside half an hour in a café, and an hour walking, all of which helps with my wellbeing.

18th January – Blean

I want to do the right things and do them correctly. Part of this entails going into school today to talk to the staff about the confirmed diagnosis and retirement. I want the staff to be the first beyond my immediate family to know my confirmed diagnosis, and to hear it from myself and not by rumour or a third party. The diagnosis was a shock to most present, but the following decision to retire was more expected. Afterwards I felt much more able to stay and chat with individuals about the situation but also to find out how they are doing both at work and outside of the school.

19th January – Blean

This evening I returned to school, this time to speak to the school governors about my diagnosis and impending retirement. This is a continuation of wanting to get this right. I feel it's important that I convey the right information to the right people at the right time. Yesterday I began this process with the staff, today it was an opportunity to speak with the governors, and then for tomorrow, I left with Lynne, the acting head, a letter to parents, which conveys much the same information to them. Hopefully the letter will be sent home at the appropriate time. I trust the staff to respect my reason for them holding onto this information for a couple of days, before the whole school community know about it.

21st January – Canterbury

This is likely to be Rosemary's last working day as a dental nurse. She's covered the role since the mid- to late 1980s, and has become a well-respected dental nurse, having previously spent many years working in an office. For the last year or two, she's been covering staff absence and not having such regular hours. It will be a new beginning for her now that she's formally retired, and will give us more time to do things together and independently.

25th January – Canterbury

We are so lucky to live close to the Hambrook Marshes, a nature reserve on our doorstep. Literally, we can see it from our lounge window, and enjoy the view when we're sitting on the patio, looking out over the river and the marshes, and watching the donkeys, sheep and chickens from the farm next door along with very vocal guinea fowl. All this within walking distance – about a mile – of Canterbury Cathedral and city centre. There is a path which goes from Canterbury out to the local villages, and it's also tarmacked so that cyclists use it. It runs alongside the River Stour and consequently is a haven for wildlife such as water birds – including egrets and herons as well as varieties of ducks and swans. As well as sitting and enjoying the ever-changing view, I do walk along the path and know it helps me keep active. I did try James's bike last week, but due to my problems with balance, it was just too difficult. I was wobbling around and I didn't feel safe. So, I'm afraid, having been a very proficient and active cyclist for a number of years, I haven't cycled for a while and am not likely to again. Clearly, it's going to be too difficult with the dementia, so walking will be my form of exercise on the track.

26th January – Shepherdswell

Rosemary and I have now joined an over-50s club in Shepherdswell, a village between Canterbury and Dover. It meets once a month, for a natter with a cup of tea, and outside speakers come in and present to us. It's a really nice social afternoon and it enables us to reconnect with folk who live in the village where we lived from 1995 to 2000. That reconnection is very important to me now that I'm retired.

27th January – Canterbury

Today I spent a lot of time phoning around to try to sort out holiday insurance for a forthcoming trip to Australia, and beyond. Because of

Alzheimer's, annual policies are now no longer available to me, so it has to be for single trips. It is interesting to see that some insurance companies wouldn't insure me because of the Alzheimer's, but thankfully some would.

1st February – Whitstable and Canterbury

Rosemary was at art class today, which allowed me to walk along the beach again at Whitstable. Now it's part of the weekly routine, and I'm really enjoying the routine, the scenery, the exercise, and listening to the music on my iPod as I walk.

The final piece in the jigsaw of my professional exit was to go to the termly head teacher meeting, which when I was on secondment I used to chair. I arranged with the person who succeeded me as Canterbury's advisor for me to have a ten-minute slot to speak with head teacher colleagues at their meeting about why I was retiring, and to say thank you and farewell to them all.

Everyone was really understanding, and lots of kind words were spoken. They knew I was going to talk about retiring but did not know the reason why. Consequently, they had all signed a card with some lovely messages. I was able to speak calmly and professionally, although did get upset afterwards in the quiet of the return home, but then I reflected upon a moving but positive conclusion to my working relationship with them all.

6th February – Canterbury

I read up on the escitalopram drug which I was prescribed a few weeks ago, and I decided to stop taking it. I'm not depressed. I'm frustrated, I'm bored, I'm unstimulated, I'm intellectually drifting, but, certainly, I'm not depressed. I need a challenge. I need a focus. I don't need a drug. Though as I said to my GP, I would welcome something to slow down what I expect to be the progression of Alzheimer's disease.

8th February – East Malling

Second and final occupational health assessment at East Malling, near Maidstone. I recounted the consultation with the neurologist, the assessments at the memory clinic, the GP's involvement, and how they're all pointing to the confirmed diagnosis of Alzheimer's disease, and the need to put into place everything that is required for me to achieve early retirement on health grounds. The professional at occupational health was very understanding, and this time, unlike the first appointment, I was very open and very transparent with them around what I was dealing with, because there was nothing to gain from withholding any information. In fact, quite the reverse. By sharing everything, it may hopefully result in a successful conclusion and a recommendation that I should retire early on the grounds of ill health (Alzheimer's), and then this door can close and I can seek another one to open. This will end this feeling of being in limbo or purgatory.

11th February – Canterbury

Discharged today from Kent and Canterbury urology department, after a couple of years of intermittent urinary tract infections. They checked the full 'waterworks' situation with me and told me that I seem to be better, and now they are prescribing tamsulosin for life. So that's one drug that I'll have to take, and I hope that it works.

13th February – Canterbury

Today I met with Gerry Warren, chief reporter from the *Kentish Gazette*, who contacted me regarding him writing an article on my diagnosis of Alzheimer's, and resultant retirement from my job as a head teacher. I've known Gerry for over 20 years from various school-related projects the local paper has covered in my role as a teacher and then as a head. He's someone I can trust, and I think I can work with. We had a constructive conversation about my story, about the diagnosis, and about my attempts to live as well as possible with dementia. He is about my age, so I got a sense from the conversation that he was relating to my experience, and I guess there was an element within his eyes of him thinking there but for the grace of God.

17th February – Canterbury

The article in the *Kentish Gazette* was published today, and with three photographs extended to a full page, which flattered me. The article is very well written, being accurate and as upbeat as possible, which pleased me. The headline 'The day I was told I had Alzheimer's' seemed a bit apocalyptic but I guess it is designed to be eye-catching.

18th February–18th March – South Australia

Four weeks of Australian sun, good friends and familiar alongside new sights has proved most restorative. All our Aussie mates know about the dementia and are most understanding and supportive. Whilst we stayed this time within South Australia, we did travel quite extensively with the support of friends to Robe in the south of the state and the Yorke Peninsula to the west. A second very successful trip after last year the neurologist saying, 'Don't go!'

21st March – Dover

I had an appointment today at Buckland Hospital, Dover, with Mr Schultz, who's an ophthalmic surgeon, because I've been referred by the optician due to a suspected problem called an epiretinal membrane, which means you've got more black floaters in front of your eyes than you should have. I seem to have loads of them at the moment, and apparently it's something that can be treated quite readily with eye drops and monitoring.

23rd March – Canterbury

A quiet day at home. The highlight for me was in the afternoon when I had a visitor come to see me, a clinical psychologist who is based in Dover, and whose name is Reinhard Guss. This is something which Elizabeth Field, who led my assessment at the memory clinic, suggested putting in place, because this guy wants to meet with me to discuss potential collaborations in the future connected to young onset dementia.

We seemed to get on pretty well in the meeting today, and it was interesting, because he lives locally to me. I understand from what he said that his wife and one of my teachers at Blean are sisters. Small world, or rather it's indicative of Canterbury as a small city. I hope that we can build upon this over the coming months, and that with his help and encouragement I will be able to put to good use some of the skills, drive and enthusiasm that I've retained, rather than sitting at home, which seems to be the order of most days at the moment.

He did also answer one of my questions, which was around which books I can read to gain more information about dementia, because I do feel at the moment that information is power, and I want to better understand what it is that I'm contending with. Alongside this, if I am to engage with and be respected by professionals, I need to do so from a position of having some greater knowledge beyond my own experience. The book that he recommended was called *Dancing with Dementia*, by an Australian called Christine Bryden. Tomorrow I'll go into Canterbury and order a copy.

28th March – Whitstable

Rosemary and I attended a post-diagnosis group meeting in a church hall in Whitstable, entitled 'Living with Dementia'. There were about eight couples there, each of whom had one person with a recent diagnosis of young onset dementia. Amongst the group was a guy called Melvyn and his wife, Jan. They're certainly two people I do remember because Melvyn was quite outspoken. I can't remember the names of many of the others, but they're all from the local area, and aged mid- to late 50s like myself, or early 60s. We had a presentation by Elizabeth Field, and a psychiatrist who was introduced as Dr Richard Brown. I said to Rosemary, 'I used to teach a Richard Brown about 22 years ago in primary school – how old do you think he is?' He heard this and said, 'Yes Mr Oliver, you were my teacher!' He then graciously came over and we spoke briefly, but then at much greater length at break time about his and my recall of each other from long ago. Amongst his memories was of me reading *The Hobbit* to the class and performing a memorable version of the voice of Gollum – many years before the Hollywood movie!

31st March – Canterbury

Michael van Stratten visited me as part of the retirement package with my union, the NAHT (National Association of Head Teachers). His job is to advise newly retired head teachers about how to invest their pension in order to make the maximum use of it. Some of his suggestions around investment are a bit ambitious for me. I'm a safe person, and I don't like taking undue risks and gambles in life, least of all with money that I cannot get again in the future. He helped also with advice about our mortgage, and he was particularly helpful around lasting power of attorney, because although I've got the forms from the Citizens Advice Bureau, I'm overwhelmed by them. I just don't know where to start. What Michael did was explain which pages to focus on, and which ones not to concern myself with. Rosemary and I are determined to do this together because we recognise its importance.

1st April – Canterbury

I retired officially today as a teacher, and as a head. Being April Fool's Day seems fitting to me because in a way some days the image of the fool is how I see myself in the future. I raised a glass to primary school heads and teachers who bravely carry the baton of putting the children first, which was always my mantra. To reinforce this, I looked again at the cards, emails and letters from Blean parents, which were most touching and really kind, supportive and humbling.

11th April – Whitstable

The second post-diagnosis meeting was very similar to the first one on 28th March: the same venue, the same people there, the same professionals speaking, and we're getting to know each other better within the group. Alongside this, there's a sense that many of us want something more as a group beyond this. We'll see. Time will tell whether that is brought into fruition.

Also, I was able to give Richard Brown an exercise book that he'd written aged ten, on a project in my class about Australia. I think this meant a great deal to him, as it did to me. My presentation of the book was done formally in front of everyone else in the group, and we all had a good laugh, which gave a nice interlude to the more serious topic of discussing dementia. Today, Richard aside, was another opportunity for me to begin to build my knowledge of dementia, which to be honest starts from a very low base.

14th April – Canterbury

I had a second meeting with Reinhard Guss, who I now refer to as Reinhard, and we agreed to meet approximately monthly. At this meeting we discussed more ideas for our future projects, so clearly there is this sense that maybe we can do something more together rather than just talk about what we might do. He told me about a horticultural project he had run with one or two colleagues in Medway quite recently, which had focused on young onset dementia. Maybe he's thinking of doing something similar down here in Canterbury, I don't know. We do share a passion for gardening, and part of our time together, as the sun was shining, was spent in my garden; this gave me a chance to show him what Rosemary and I had set out to try to achieve in the garden. Reinhard told me about his love of gardening too. Good to have common ground there beyond the discussion around dementia. I feel that's important if we are going to do something together in the future, that he gets to know me as a person, and similarly, I hope that I get to know him as a person as well, whilst maintaining that professional respect which he and his role deserve.

15th April – Canterbury

I met a lovely person named Judy Ayris from Canterbury Age Concern. She came to see Rosemary and me, and I get a sense that she's going to be a great ally in the future. She came across as really bubbly, very kind and clearly thoughtful. She knew what she was talking about, and was a great encourager of looking at what practical help there might be out there for us. Judy left with us some forms to fill in, and said she would come back in a couple of weeks to collect them.

Judy also sensed that I want to know more about dementia, so she recommended *Person-Centred Counselling for People with Dementia* by an author named Danuta Lipinska, which I will also seek to get.

Finally, when she was about to leave, she talked to us a little bit about a unit at Age Concern for younger people with dementia, called the Collins Unit, and she encouraged Rosemary and me to come in and have a look on Wednesday, to see whether we think it might be some use to me now or in the future.

16th April – Canterbury

We had a really interesting evening last night, which is unusual, because these days…I wouldn't say I don't go out in the evening, but I don't go out very much, and last night, Rosemary and I went for a dusk bat walk over on the marshes with a guide, and electronic bat detectors. Despite being free it was really poorly supported. I suppose there were about four or five people there. We did detect lots of different bats including pipistrelle and long eared, zooming over the surface of the river catching flies and insects and then feeding their offspring clinging precariously to the Victorian brickwork of the underside of a railway bridge. Yet another example of our good fortune to live close to nature.

20th April – Canterbury

We visited the Collins Unit for young onset dementia at Canterbury Age Concern. It's not for me at the moment. It really is for people with more advanced dementia, but at least I've had a look, and now I've been inside Age Concern and I know where the building is alongside some of the other activities they offer.

I finished reading *Dancing with Dementia* by Christine Bryden. It was far more helpful to me than *My Bonnie*, the book by John Suchet that I read last year. I found it really honest, constructive, and the true experience of someone living with young onset dementia. *My Bonnie* was an interesting read, and it told the story of the disease through the eyes of John Suchet, who is a carer, and is basically a love story, and it is in many senses a story of loss. I found it a bit depressing, really, if I'm going to be honest. This is the first time I have read an account by a carer. I offered it to Rosemary, and Rosemary certainly didn't want to read it, and I can understand that. But with *Dancing with Dementia*, the title says it all, and I got a lot of encouragement from the book and feel reading it is a potential turning point for me.

21st April – Canterbury

Rick Harris, a researcher from Customer Faithful, who are sponsored by Dementia UK and Pfizer, came to see me today to talk about my views on having dementia, alongside my views on medication for dementia, and what I would feel could be helpful to allow me to live well in the period soon after being diagnosed. I am one of six people from three European countries to be interviewed. This is the first professional from outside of our local area to visit me, and to involve me in a piece of research. This all seems so alien and strange to me alongside a simmering sense of doing something useful once again with my life.

22nd April – Fordwich

Fordwich is where we lived from 1981 to 1995. It is the smallest town in Britain, situated three miles outside Canterbury. Rosemary and I walked past our old house, then along the Stour Valley Walk which passed through our former garden up into the nearby woods where we were greeted by a profuse carpet of blue, as the bluebells were in full flower. The scents and the sights were magnificent. A magical moment to savour the present, to take solace in the moment and connect back to our past memories.

27th April – Canterbury

Because I miss the children at school, I've had a conversation recently with Clive Close, the head teacher of Wincheap School near to where I live, and a head I know well. Clive and I share similar ideas on education, and on life. We put our heads together, and we've come up with a plan supported by a couple of his teachers for me to go into the school once a week on a Wednesday, to hear children read from about 9 a.m. until about 10.30. I'm really looking forward to this. The children will be eight- and nine-year-olds, and there will be about six to eight of them. I am really pleased to be able to contribute, and bring something back to a school and to children for as long as I'm able to.

Before I left the school at the end of the session, Clive stopped me and I had a long conversation with him about how life is treating me, how welcoming the teachers had been, and the encouragement I'd felt from the morning with the children.

29th April – Canterbury

Royal wedding day. I didn't really want to be involved in watching Kate and William, but actually it became quite addictive. Our next-door neighbours, Jean and Andy, came round, and we had a bacon brunch with champagne with them whilst watching the procession and ceremony. Whilst Andy and I weren't keen at the start, we got hooked by the ladies' enthusiasm, and I guess by the pageantry and the spectacle of the event.

4th May – Canterbury

Went for an MRI scan again, one year on from the last one. This was a suggestion by me to Elizabeth Field and Mary Aston, who commissioned it with the Kent and Canterbury Hospital. I do sense a decline, and I want to know what's happening in my brain.

5th May – Canterbury

I am finding it disconcerting now that when travelling in the car as a passenger I do not register seeing things outside which Rosemary points out to me.

As part of our membership of the U3A, today we went on a historic walk around the city. Similar to my sense of living near the marshes, the outskirts of Canterbury are a really wonderful place to live, and to be able to access the history of this city is a real treat. History has always been a big love of mine, and whilst I don't read as much now because I can't remember what I'm reading, I never tire of living in a city where I can see history around every corner.

11th May – Ashford

Today I attended my first peer support group being run by the Alzheimer's Society in Ashford. I'd arranged it with Ellie from the Alzheimer's Society, as there's nothing more local to where I live. It's a well-established group of older-onset people, with the diagnosed person and their family carer attending for half a day. I was really pleased about managing the train journey and the walk from the station to the venue on my own. I had three different maps with me, and two different copies of timetables, so I was very well prepared, which gave me the extra confidence to be able to do this. I also rang Rosemary three times during the morning – on the journey, at the place and on the way back – so that both our minds were put at ease that I was safe.

21st May – Canterbury

A lovely warm, sunny day to coincide with the official opening of the Kingfisher Way, which is the name given to the path that runs through the Hambrook Marshes from Canterbury, past our house, out to the village of Chartham. It was lovely to be able to support something which gives us so much pleasure and restorative energy.

23rd May – Sturry

We attended the first meeting of a young onset support group which is more local to us. The meeting was held in a pub in Sturry on the outskirts of Canterbury and organised by a new charity called EKIDS (East Kent Independent Dementia Support). I understand they are a group of people who formerly were part of the Alzheimer's Society, but for one reason or another have now set up their own small charity independent of that big organisation.

Membership of this support group was open to those who were part of the post-diagnostic group which met a few months ago. Many of us wanted to stay together and were then introduced to EKIDS by the memory clinic, who have taken over the responsibility of coordinating this. It's run as a dementia café, where we sit and have sandwiches and a cup of tea, chat and find out what support, if any, is going to be available to us. We all plan to now meet once a month.

We also talked about having trips as a group, which will be a positive thing to do because we all get on quite well as a group of people drawn together by young onset dementia.

24th May – Blean

I went back into school to celebrate my retirement, first of all with the children in a special assembly, and then after school with a special tea with the staff, governors and representatives from the local authority. I wrote a poem to read to the children about moving on through life, and the head boy and head girl prepared a 'Parkinson style' interview with me which we did as a part of the assembly. The hymn I chose seemed fitting on many levels – once again 'One More Step Along the World I Go' – and the music for the children to enter and leave by was Andrea Bocelli and Sarah Brightman singing 'Time to Say Goodbye'. My emotions were a mixture of sadness to be leaving the wonderful staff and children, a sense of a job done as well as I could over the past 11 years, and relief that it was over and that the closure went as well as it did.

26th May – Canterbury

Slept better after a poor previous night. I suspect the events at school were subconsciously playing on my mind and awakened me at 4 a.m., after which I could not go back to sleep. Despite this, Rosemary and I participated in the U3A treasure hunt around the city, and we won it! There were 25 couples taking part, and I kept it secret that the guy with his wife who had won this competition had Alzheimer's! This thought made me smile afterwards.

28th May – Canterbury

The *Kentish Gazette* published a piece again about me, Gerry having visited me to do a follow-up article to the one he wrote a few months ago, this time focusing on the actual retirement event that took place at school. The headline this time was a moving 'We'll all miss you Mr Oliver!' The piece included a splendid photograph, of me at my leaving assembly with all 460 children in the background. I feel my smile in the photograph, and the piece Gerry wrote conveyed all the right messages.

4th–6th June – Nottingham

We travelled to Nottingham to see my mum in her care home.

She did remember me, which is always a relief. My mother has Alzheimer's, and it has become more advanced quite rapidly. She's now totally immobile and needs a hoist to be moved, so consequently she doesn't drink enough, because unsurprisingly she hates being lifted in this hoist to be put in a wheelchair in order to go to the toilet. Then she gets dehydrated, leading to various infections, all of which add to her challenges.

The care home is quite a good one, and they do genuinely, I think, care for her, but she's bored. Like many others she's sitting there not doing very much, and when I go and see her our time together is probably one of the most stimulating times of her week or month.

She did remember, also, to tell me off, as her Mother's Day card, which she still had displayed by her chair in the lounge, had 'mother' on it rather than 'mam'. I tried in vain to explain that you can't get a card that says 'mam' on it in Canterbury! This northern expression is not used down here, but she has never accepted this as a reason or excuse.

Her view is, once a 'mam', always a 'mam'.

She also often talked about my father, and asked when he's coming to see her. I have to be honest with her, but also I don't want to hurt her, and cause her to grieve again. She did attend his funeral, and that was a very traumatic experience for her, and for others because of that. What I say to her, which seems to pacify her, is 'He's not coming today.' I know it's perfectly truthful – he isn't coming today, of course, nor tomorrow, nor any other day, because he passed away in 2010.

7th June – Canterbury

I had my six-monthly check with Dr Aston at the memory clinic today. Maybe I think too much, but I have always been a deep thinker, and I will try and work out how to deal with the ups and downs that dementia is presenting me with. Dr Aston sensitively gave me feedback on the scan I had in May, and explained to me that there had been little change, except that the hippocampus had shrunk a little, and there was a bit more atrophy in certain parts of the brain. I asked if I could have a copy of the scan, and she advised that I could, and that the cost would be £25, which I duly paid; I will get a copy of the scan in a week or so. I'm not sure that I could understand it, or indeed whether I would spend time looking at it – it just seemed something I wanted to have.

10th June – Canterbury

Had a visit today from Daren Kerle, who is a community officer at Canterbury City Library. Daren had read the articles about me in the local paper, and he came to discuss with me whether I was happy to do some voluntary work with him in the library on a project called Read Aloud. This involves folk who are in the mid- to late stages of Alzheimer's or other dementias in reading profusely illustrated books with their loved ones, or having loved ones look at the book with them and chat about the memories that the text and pictures evoke. I felt I could relate to Daren and the project so it could be another 'thing to get my teeth into'.

14th June – Canterbury

Sinead McGettrick, the Admiral Nurse, met Rosemary at Morrisons café for a follow-up to her first visit last December, this time without me. Rosemary is not too keen on seeing Sinead, because she feels that there are more needy folk who need to access her more than she does, but she knows that Sinead is there for her if and when required. I didn't question Rosemary afterwards about the meeting she had. Knowing how sensitive we are to each other's feelings, snippets will come out in conversation when we each feel comfortable with sharing.

18th–25th June – Scotland

Great to visit Scotland for the first time, but gee it is such a long way by coach and I am exhausted. We don't think we will ever do a coach tour such as this again.

27th June – Canterbury

Still feeling tired after our trip but visited at my home by Penny Hibberd, who is the director of the dementia centre at Canterbury Christ Church

University. She had met me at the Ashford dementia group and asked me to help with a project in testing out a tracker device. Today she brought an engineer with her, from the company making the tracker phone device, to talk about my views on this piece of equipment.

I have to say, trialling this over the past two weeks was a mixed experience. I was pleased to try it, because I feel that technologies such as this can be useful in helping people with dementia maintain their independence, but in conversation with John, the engineer, I got the sense that they wanted an endorsement, and not constructively critical suggestions which is what I thought would be more useful to them.

The device had worked accurately 75 per cent of the time, though one time I was on Whitstable beach, and it placed me about a mile away on the high street, which was of concern if I was requiring help.

29th June – Maidstone

I went with Reinhard to Maidstone to speak to the KMPT NHS Trust board. Talk about being thrown in at the deep end for your first encounter with the world of dementia management. I was very nervous travelling up in Reinhard's car and chatted away all the time in monologue mode! Once there the chairman and Reinhard's boss were most welcoming and friendly and put me at ease. The 15 minutes with them flew by and I am told it is the first time many of them had met someone with dementia and that I had made a very positive and useful impact, all of which has given me a confidence boost to do more if possible.

5th July – Canterbury

I am pleased to be starting to take galantamine (Reminyl), an anti-Alzheimer's medication. The initial strength of dose is 8 mg. I've been feeling very tired recently, so it will be interesting to see how I fare with these tablets.

13th–14th July – Canterbury

Attended my first dementia conference at Canterbury Christ Church University. Rosemary came with me for day one, and I went on my own for day two.

I don't remember a lot about the conference, thinking back now on the evening of the 14th, but what I do remember is, on the second day, I had written down to attend a circle dance workshop. This was because the after-lunch options were a talk about end of life (I certainly didn't want to go to that), caring for someone with dementia (with a primary target audience of carers), and a light-hearted practical workshop entitled 'circle dance'. Well, I'm hopeless at dancing, but I thought that was the least bad of the three options.

I decided this morning to take a book with me and thought I may well just skive off from that session, and find a quiet space to sit and read. However, as I was going to lunch my conscience was burning in my mind, and I thought, 'I can't do that, that's wrong.' I will go into this session, and I'll sit near the door, and if it gets a bit heavy, or I feel embarrassed, I'll nip out.

Well, Celia, the person leading the workshop, who is the country's leading advocate for circle dancing, spotted the look on my face and guessed what I was thinking, so she shifted me from that seat to one furthest away from the door where there was certainly no escape.

In the room there were about 14 people: 12 women, one other chap and me. I was the only person there with dementia, as far as I know. Well, I had a hoot. It was a lovely hour, and I really did enjoy it. This experience reminds me, as I write my diary today, not to pre-judge something. Try something, and if you don't like it, well, you don't have to do it again, but at least give something a go on that first occasion. I've always tried to do that, but in the last year or so, I've tended to play safe. Today I moved away from playing safe, and it worked really well.

18th July – Faversham

Another aspect of our membership of the University of the Third Age is visiting open gardens. We love seeing what can be achieved with money and space in large gardens. A nice, leisurely afternoon with like-minded mature folk away from dealing with dementia.

We really enjoyed this afternoon, and there was a cup of tea and a lovely piece of cake to make it even better. The group meets once a month from March through to September.

25th July – Canterbury

Saw Dr Aston at the memory clinic regarding a medication check. Today she wanted to know how I was coping with galantamine. I told her absolutely fine. I don't notice, to be honest, any significant improvement, but also it's not giving me any nasty side effects and the tiredness seems a bit less noticeable. In these appointments I am cautious about what I say about how I feel in front of Rosemary as I do not want to worry her unduly, and if I do it challenges my ability to remain positive.

Psychologically, I feel a bit lifted that at last I am receiving something tangible designed to slow down the dementia.

2nd August – London

As part of Rosemary's birthday present from our eldest son Gareth and his family, we had tickets to go and see *War Horse* at the New London Theatre, plus a lovely afternoon tea at Fortnum and Mason's. She really did feel 'like the bee's knees'. It was a real treat. I had read the book *War Horse*, and found it really good, but the show was outstanding. Absolutely outstanding. In fact, Michael Morpurgo, the author, and I met about two or three years ago when I was participating in a head teacher conference, and he was the keynote speaker, talking about education and children which are genuine passions of his. Coincidentally, in his early 20s, he taught in a primary school in Wickhambreaux, which is a small village just outside Canterbury, and as a child he was a pupil at King's School in Canterbury. Michael and I had a conversation about Canterbury, and about Wickhambreaux, and subsequent to that, I put him in touch with the head teacher who's currently leading that school. Michael went back to visit the school, and unveiled a plaque to mark the opening of a new classroom building.

3rd August – Fordwich

Today was another return to our old stamping ground, this time with the family history group for a convivial lunch in the local pub. Whilst the focus is family history, the group are such interesting people that we do diverge from that, and talk about life in general. We are beginning to forge good friendships within the group, and it's a constructive diversion from groups like the EKIDS group, where the main focus is dementia.

6th August – Herne Bay

I was pleased it was a warm sunny day for our first EKIDS outing, which was a white-knuckle ride for me in a speedboat out into the Thames estuary to visit the Maunsell Forts and the Kent wind farm. I thought a short-sleeved shirt seemed the right attire for this dalliance with the jet set. Rosemary, thankfully, convinced me to take a cagoule just in case. Once we were out on the sea, WOW, the wind got up, and the sea became very choppy, very grey and very cold for a formerly warm August afternoon. The speedboat was racing through the water and bouncing up and down, so consequently, I was clinging on to the rope that was next to me where I was seated. Only afterwards did I notice that my knuckles were raw and bleeding. Apart from that, it was a really good day! Rosemary and the EKIDS chair decided that they wouldn't venture into the boat, and they spent the hour or two we were out on the sea in a café nearby. I'm not sure which was the best of the two options!

9th–14th August – Nottingham and Crewe

Five-hundred-mile round trip to visit my mother in her care home and Brian, our close family friend from Crewe. Both of them are living in very different circumstances but are keeping quite well.

24th August – Canterbury

Dominic McCully, our solicitor, visited us today to confirm with us our lasting power of attorney which we've written, and to help update our wills, or more accurately, write our wills, because we previously wrote them when I was 25, back in 1981 when we got married, and clearly they needed revising. With Dominic's assistance today, we completed setting in place our wishes for the future. I asked Dominic to include a clause in my will to state that it is my wish that when I die my ashes are taken by one of our children and scattered under a eucalypt tree in Australia. This has given us peace of mind, knowing that we've addressed the power of attorney and our wills and they can now be 'parked' until required.

25th August – Canterbury

I have now finished reading the book *Losing Clive to Younger Onset Dementia*, written by Helen Beaumont. The book is about an ex-soldier who developed young onset dementia in his 40s, and died from it just a few years later. His wife, Helen Beaumont, wrote the book as a tribute, and as a way of sharing his account with the world. Helen felt that young onset dementia was poorly understood and that there was no support for those living with it. To try and address this she established the Clive Project in Oxford. I will now go online and find out what I can draw from this.

8th September – Medway

I attended a conference today organised by Penny Hibberd at Christchurch University in Chatham, to discuss assistive technology. Penny invited Rosemary and me along to talk about the phone tracker that I trialled a few months ago. Penny also passed over to me a copy of a book called *Still Alice*, which looks interesting. I've taken it to read and will return it to her with some feedback. It's a novel written by Lisa Genova about a woman who was a university lecturer in America, who developed young onset dementia in her early–mid 50s. As I've just finished reading a book I am keen to start this one tonight.

16th September – Canterbury

Reinhard visited for our seventh monthly meeting, and this time, he brought along with him a young placement student named Ian who is working with the Kent and Medway Partnership Trust for a year as part of his psychology degree course. Ian seems like a really friendly, able young man. He comes from Wakefield, in Yorkshire, and is really into rugby league. Ian's passionate about completing his degree and going on to work with people with dementia as a clinical psychologist. If I can help with that in any way, then I'd be only too happy to do so as it allows me to reconnect to my former role in helping support and nurture young students and professionals entering a caring profession.

Investing in the future generation has been and still is a key focus for me. I was thinking about this when walking along the beach at Whitstable recently – often the site of my best thinking. I understand that under tall trees saplings do struggle to grow, but it is also foolish to expect an acorn planted in the morning to be an oak tree by evening. In other words, bringing out the best in others is an art and a skill and takes time to nurture and support.

I have identified three possible approaches to living with dementia: give up; sit back and avoid it and live life as if it doesn't exist; or confront it and do something about it – I am going for the third option!

24th September – Whitstable and Canterbury

Following the visit from Daren, the librarian, I attended a Read Aloud meeting to help as a volunteer with the use of picture books for people with more advanced dementia and carers. Connected to this, I delivered a talk afterwards to library staff who had been invited to hear about what living with dementia is like for me, and how that contrasts, but runs parallel to, the five or six people with dementia who were participants in today's session, each of whom are much further into their dementia than I am, and in all cases much older.

I saw Dr Aston at the Canterbury memory clinic, and she increased my galantamine to 16 mg because I'm experiencing no problems with the lower dose. I now understand that I'm on the middle dose, because it goes 8 mg, 16 mg, and then the maximum is 24 mg. I want to try and hold off from the maximum for as long as I possibly can, so I can have that in reserve for when it's required.

25th September – Whitstable

I participated in the Alzheimer's Society's annual memory walk today, which took us from Whitstable Castle, down along the seafront, up as far as Swalecliffe, a suburb of Whitstable where I was deputy head back in the 1990s, and then back along the seafront. There were between 80 and 100 people walking, virtually all of them carers and former carers. I wasn't aware of anyone else with a diagnosis of dementia there. Also walking were a number of students who were interested in being involved and supporting the event, plus a smattering of people from the community, who thought that this was a cause that they wanted to support.

I personally raised £350 for the Alzheimer's Society from friends, family and generous support from Wincheap School and from my former colleagues back at Blean. It was a lovely sunny day. The lord mayor and local celebrity Janet Street-Porter said a few words at the beginning, cut the ribbon, and then launched the walk before going off to other events that they needed to attend to, leaving the walkers to amble along, and enjoy conversations as we strolled.

The organisers had arranged for me to walk with a lovely volunteer student from the University of Kent. I can't remember her name, but she was a really pleasant young person, very engaging, very good conversationalist, and the walk whizzed by because of the time we spent chatting. I suppose we were walking for about 50 minutes. Rosemary waved me off at the start, went for a coffee, and then met me at the end.

1st October – London
Greater investment into dementia research is essential, and allied to this I am taking advantage of an opportunity to join the Alzheimer's Society Research Network as a volunteer. Today's training event for new volunteers took place at Asthma UK because they and the Alzheimer's Society pool their resources to train volunteers in scientific research. Half of the day we were all together, those linked to the Alzheimer's Society and those who were supporting Asthma UK, and the other half we were separate, in separate rooms, where we were able to focus on the particular health condition we were living with or working with. I also met a member of the Alzheimer's Society staff named Matt Murray, who manages the Research Network. Matt came over as a friendly person who I hope to be able to work well with in the future.

After the training workshop, Rosemary and I had arranged to meet Amanda Drury and her husband, along with their two children, by the London Eye. Amanda is a really interesting person from my past. She was one of the children I taught in a class back in Adelaide in 1989, and had gone on to spend some time in England as a primary school teacher. She told me in an email after we'd made contact that one reason she'd become a teacher was because of the inspiration I gave her to take that route.

We spent a lovely hour or so chatting away, and I took some photographs with me to share with her and her family from the time when she was in my Year 5 class. Her children were thrilled to see their mum in these old school photographs and it was great to reconnect with her after all this time, and to acknowledge and see what a really lovely person she'd grown into, and what a splendid mum she is to their two children.

8th–15th October – Italy
We had wanted a more restful holiday after Scotland and we achieved this with a week in a village close to Salerno overlooking the Bay of Naples. Flying from Manston near Ramsgate was so easy and the trip enabled us to

visit Pompeii – fascinating; the Amalfi coast – beautiful though frightening from the bus, although less so viewed from a boat; and Capri – expensive and we thought overrated.

20th October – Medway

I went with Rosemary to the Canterbury Christ Church University site at Chatham to speak to a group of healthcare students following an invitation from Penny Hibberd. I gave a summary of what living with dementia is like alongside my views on what services perhaps should be provided to people like myself. Rosemary joined me for the session and the Q&A which followed. I felt relaxed in this environment but the questions were rather uncomfortable for Rosemary. The students were asking her about how she felt about her husband having dementia. Her honest response was that it was too difficult for her to talk about. I fully respect this and will do everything to avoid her being upset in this way again.

27th October – Canterbury

Dominic, our solicitor, revisited us to confirm our wills. This time, Rosemary and I had invited along two friends from Shepherdswell who had asked to find out more about writing their wills. Neither of them have dementia, but both of them are in their late 70s, early 80s, so it seemed an appropriate time to give them access to a solicitor who may be able to advise, and not charge them a fortune.

28th October – Canterbury

There's so much to learn about our historic city, but I am increasingly frustrated that I'm starting to struggle to concentrate in talks such as this U3A one today at the city's Baptist church. Consequently, I have to make lots of notes, otherwise I don't remember anything other than where I've been, and maybe who I've been with.

8th November – Margate

Between 7th and 9th November, we had two Australian visitors stay with us, Jan and Wayne. They're amongst our network of friends from Adelaide, and because Jan is a volunteer guide at the Adelaide art gallery she really wanted to visit the Turner Gallery of Contemporary Art as it has attracted some attention in Adelaide. We all felt that the location of the gallery is splendid. It's right on the beach in Margate, and the building is impressive, but actually – appreciating that art is subjective – we all felt there wasn't a lot of quality artwork from our perspective within the gallery, so we were a little bit disappointed about the contents.

13th–18th November – Port Isaac, Cornwall

I'm writing this in my diary on 18th November, having just arrived home from five really excellent days with our dear Aussie mates Julie and Paul Reece in Port Isaac. We stayed in a cottage two or three doors away from the very building that was used as the location of Doc Martin's surgery in the TV show. We're thankful that it was November and not August when we visited, because the village is beautiful and quiet this time of year, and we were able to gain easy access to pubs and restaurants, and whatever else was available to us, without the crowds that in summer throng the incredibly narrow streets of this picturesque fishing port.

21st November – Canterbury

Dr Aston, my psychiatrist, has moved on to another post within Kent, and consequently, this was my first appointment with senior consultant Dr Beats. She focused upon checking how I was with my medication. Dr Beats seems very pleasant. I'm not sure what she and I learned from the appointment, other than that the medication is not giving me any nasty side effects and might be helping me.

23rd November – Nottingham

Travelled to attend my Auntie Maisie's funeral today. Maisie is the last member of my dad's generation. There were ten siblings in their family, and Maisie and my father were the two youngest. I attended with Rosemary, and spent some time with my cousin Jane, and Ian her husband. It was lovely to reconnect with Jane about three years ago, having had not a falling out at all, but simply a divergence of experience, whereby our paths didn't cross. There was no contact between us from 1977 to 2010. That makes me sad. I'm very sorry about that, but both of us are determined that in whatever time we have available to us, we will make sure that we do keep in contact and we'll see each other from time to time, despite the fact that her mum has now died, and my dad has also relatively recently died. Maisie was a great support to my father in his latter days, and really helped look after him in the months before his death when his health declined quite rapidly.

We also called into the home to see my mother but she was slumped asleep and sadly was not able to respond very much. The staff were firm that she shouldn't be disturbed as it might distress her, and whilst keen to see and speak with her I was resigned to respect their view and we left.

29th November – London

My first experience of the DAA (Dementia Action Alliance) is their annual conference which I attended with Ian and with Reinhard. I enjoyed the conference and the trip up to London which are new experiences to me. When I was working, trips to London were a rarity. I might go up there once or twice a year, and then possibly a similar number of times for recreational purposes. I don't know how often opportunities will arise now that I have dementia.

One thing I do remember from today is a conversation Ian and I had on the train coming back, when he pointed out to me an incident which had occurred with a civil servant from the Department of Health, who was talking to Ian, myself and a number of other people, quite openly, and quite informally. We were all engaged in the conversation, then about halfway through, we each outlined what role we were occupying. I explained that I had dementia. Ian fed back to me afterwards that the civil servant's manner and body language completely changed towards me, and there was no further interaction from him towards me after that point. I hadn't picked that up. It had gone over my head, and I'm probably thankful that it did.

It's interesting that Ian spotted this, and I'll be mindful of this in future, if I attend further meetings of this sort.

9th December – Herne Bay

Psychologist Elizabeth Field took me today to the Living with Dementia group for young onset dementia, similar to the one I attended back in the spring with Rosemary. This time I was there to speak about being positive with dementia, and trying to encourage those who were there to seek help, to develop certain strategies that I shared with them, and to try and live each day as it comes. They were the main messages I expressed alongside practical help. This was well received, and attendees' comments afterwards were most generous.

One family that were particularly interesting were a traveller family. There wasn't just the guy with dementia and his wife, or his partner, there were six people from the extended family present.

It seems ages ago since Rosemary and I were part of a group of this sort, but really a number of things have happened in that time, and my memory of events is getting vaguer.

13th December – Canterbury

Rosemary and I attended an evening talk by Reinhard about the brain at Canterbury Christ Church University, where he described with a PowerPoint presentation the functions of the brain, the processes of the brain, how the brain influences behaviour, and how professionals should seek to help people with dementia to maintain their personhood.

This is the first in-depth talk I had heard about how the brain works, and the first time I'd heard Reinhard outside of chatting to him either in our lounge, or on the two journeys we'd made together, once to Maidstone and once to London.

25th December – Canterbury

All the family converged on us and we had a lovely Christmas. We also used the opportunity to bring our three adult children more fully into the picture regarding wills and power of attorney.

31st December – Canterbury

The final pro forma for a project that Ian, Reinhard and I are working on is completed! We're looking at developing a piece of work tracking and analysing one person (i.e. me) throughout the year after being diagnosed with Alzheimer's. To do this I have completed over 40 pro formas which we had devised, outlining a range of activities which I've undertaken. Approximately half of them are dementia related, and approximately half of them are not.

All of those pro formas are now with Ian to analyse and process, using something called IPA (not Indian Pale Ale, I'm assured, but interpretive phenomenological analysis), which he has tried patiently to explain to me a number of times. He will draw conclusions around one person's attempt to live as well as possible for that first year after the diagnosis.

We have examined in depth the positive and the negative impacts of the activities, which include attending meetings, giving talks, holidays, Christmas, reading, cinema visits, gardening, using the tracker, hearing children read – there's many more, as you can imagine, making up that 40-plus list.

We now aim to try to present this at the Alzheimer's Disease International conference, which I'm told is happening in London in the spring of 2012. This will be a joint presentation between Ian, Reinhard and myself, and will draw conclusions and make recommendations to professionals, service users, carers and supporters. This is the first time since retiring that I have had something constructive outside of the home to look forward to and I am excited by the prospect.

Sometime in 2011

Dear Alzheimer's

It is now a year since my last letter to you, during which time we have had a number of encounters with each other. I sense you see this as a conflict; if so, some battles I have won, and in some you have gained an upper hand, but although your victories will leave a bitter taste, they will be short-lived.

You tried to tempt me with the falsehood that retirement would be cosy, but warning signals about boredom flashed in front of me. I know you encourage apathy, and then use this as a weapon to bring about decline. I will contest this with you through remaining busy, active, engaged and involved in projects and challenges I have enjoyed for some time alongside new ones.

Often you will hear people asking me, 'What is it like to have dementia?' You will know that I liken your influence to the weather, and when I am feeling well the sun shines brightly and you flee into the darkness; when you are most active the fog descends either in patches or as an impenetrable shroud. You will also have heard me say that on the foggy days, tomorrow will be better and the sun will reappear. The other image I use is of a picture which a hole punch has made holes in, sometimes few, sometimes many. If it's the latter then the sheet is discarded and a new picture emerges to restore my confidence and help me move forward.

Paramount in my mind at this time is my desire to establish a new life which maintains what you are seeking to take from me, which is my identity, my personhood, my place in the world, my humanity. All of these at this time are well out of your reach, although I do sense you stretching out your grasping hands to wrench them from me. You have few allies and mine are growing in number. Unlike you, I am not alone, I have others helping me to surround myself with a protective shell.

Never truly yours

Keith

2012

—

'Envoy'

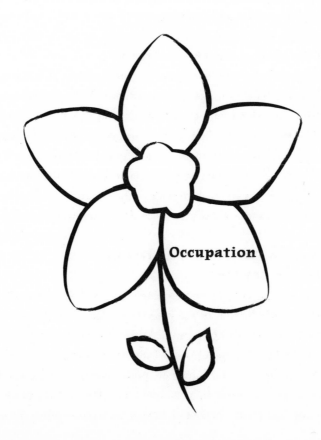

Occupation

4th January – Canterbury

A new year begins with meeting Ian Asquith to discuss his placement project. It's good to reunite with Ian again after the Christmas break and it's given me food for thought around the importance of education which, for me, was free, and was my escape from what could have been a lifetime working in a factory or an office. I had an interview when I was 16 at Boots, and really wanted a clerical job there as I hated Years 10 and 11 at school doing my O levels, and wanted to leave. I'm so thankful that I didn't get the job, and that I went on to do A levels and then went to university. Education serves to raise your aspirations and extends opportunities – it certainly did this for me.

6th January – Canterbury

I have just finished reading a book about Tom Kitwood. What I took from it was that care plans should be about what the person *can* do, rather than what they previously could do and cannot do any more – if only I had a care plan!

18th January–2nd March – Australia

A six-week trip to Australia to escape the British winter. A bonus of being retired and a real boost to us both. Time with dear Alan and Glenys relaxing, eating, drinking and swimming with friends (and a visiting dolphin!) were the highlights of the first half of our trip before heading off with Bev and John to enjoy their company in their gorgeous beach home on the Yorke Peninsula. Even though we no longer venture far from Adelaide, our favourite location has so much to offer in the summer sunshine to satisfy our hearts, minds and souls. Maybe again next year – we hope so!

7th, 9th, 10th March – ADI conference, ExCeL Centre, London

Refreshed from our holiday and looking back on three jam-packed days which were a culmination of the project Ian, Reinhard and I had been working on for a number of months. We'd been granted a poster at the prestigious ADI (Alzheimer's Disease International) conference in London. Half of the time was spent manning our poster, meeting people, and talking about our project, supported by a handout based closely on the poster which we gave out. The poster looked at service user involvement from three perspectives: that of the service user, the professional and the supporter, who in this case was Ian, supporting as a student.

Also during the conference, we were able to access some really excellent talks, and to begin what I recognise is the process of networking, largely through Reinhard, who introduced us to a number of his friends and colleagues.

Ian and I travelled up and back each day in his car. On the evening of the 7th there was a drinks event to launch the conference, during which people like Terry Pratchett were in attendance, and Ian photographed me alongside the great man. Apart from Ian, I didn't know anybody there. What it did serve to do was to give me an opportunity to meet Gaynor Smith, who works for the Alzheimer's Society. I gave Gaynor really negative feelings around the support that I had received thus far from the Alzheimer's Society. This is largely due to the fact that, in East Kent, there is very little presence from the society. Rather than feel upset by this and walk off with her tail between her legs, Ian spotted Gaynor moving over towards the posters, which were nearby, and to focus on the one that we had created. Clearly, some impact was made on her, and likewise, her doing this created a very positive impression upon me.

12th March – Maidstone

I went to the KMPT Young Onset Dementia conference with Reinhard and Ian yesterday. I spoke to a large healthcare audience about my experience of living with young onset dementia, and made recommendations to professionals in order to improve the services available within Kent. First of all, I focused on people being true to themselves, both as professionals, and as people going through the process of being diagnosed, and then moving into the post-diagnosis phase. I spoke in depth about things that I am currently involved in supporting within Kent, and I used the phrase 'service users should always do their very best to focus on what they can do, rather than what they can't do'. Also by implication this is equally relevant to professionals.

13th March – Canterbury

This morning I gave a talk to healthcare students at Canterbury Christ Church University. The focus was a reflection upon the onset of my dementia, and how it crept up on me. I explained my diagnosis in depth, about how I'd gone through the GP, and then the neurologist, and finally ended up at the memory clinic in Canterbury. I concluded by explaining the book *The Seven Habits of Highly Effective People* by Stephen R. Covey, introduced to me by spinal specialist Christian Farthing, and how important the circles of influence and concern are in managing one's life. The circle of influence is at the centre, where we place things where we can actually make a difference. Surrounding that is the circle of concern. That's things which have an impact upon us. We should try if we possibly can to extend the circle of influence in order to exert some control over those concerns. Everything else should be parked outside of those two circles. I wish I had known about this when I was working.

Alongside that, I spoke to them about the importance of interdependence, i.e. communicating with other people and continuing to stay connected, and independence, which would mean being able to function on one's own. Both are important, but often professionals overlook the former and concentrate solely on the latter, which to me can mean being isolated and lonely.

20th March – Canterbury

My annual dementia check with the GP. He checked my blood pressure, we had a chat but little more really, and I'm not sure how useful it was, other than to keep me on his radar. I also got the sense that perhaps he was fulfilling a requirement rather than producing something constructive for either of us.

Following the GP appointment, I have been with Ian to speak at the Psychology Society at Kent University. There were about 15 students in attendance, all members of the Psychology Society. I found them friendly and interested. Ian had helped me with preparation, and I was able to talk about the symptoms of dementia, focusing on mine alongside giving them the general picture and how the two sat alongside each other. I spoke about the diagnosis, and how I was able to cope with dementia, illustrating this partly by the metaphors of the weather – the foggy days and the sunny days – and then followed that with the image of a swan being serene and fairly calm, and presenting in a certain way on the surface, but below the surface paddling sometimes more madly depending on which direction the current is flowing.

23rd–26th March – Weymouth

A welcome change of scenery with Rosemary, joining her Women's Institute (WI) group travelling to Weymouth for a few days. The sun shone, both weather-wise and healthwise, and it was a lovely little break down there, with a group of approximately 50 to 60 senior citizens who are members of the Shepherdswell Women's Institute and their husbands.

28th March – Canterbury

Having first read *Dancing with Dementia* 11 months ago I decided to re-read it and this time to make notes to help me remember some passages. It is such an important book.

Following on from the previous article a year ago, Gerry Warren from the *Kentish Gazette* newspaper called in today on a prearranged visit to speak to me, and then write up a follow-up piece about how I am coping with Alzheimer's. I am not quite sure what he expected to find – maybe he was surprised that I haven't slipped into the realms of 'the only just with us brigade'!

1st–3rd April – Nottingham

Just arrived back in Canterbury from visiting my mother in Nottingham. She was generally in quite good form. She still recognises me and Rosemary, despite her advancing Alzheimer's, although she is now totally immobile so there's no opportunities to take her out. She continues to require a hoist to lift her out of her seat in order to go to the toilet, or to do anything beyond sitting in the lounge. The time spent with her was mostly me talking; to support this we took some photos along to show her. Many of the residents who share the home with her are more advanced in their dementia, although I suspect that she perks up because we are with her and she is engaged and happy. My mother does not, and will not, know that I also have Alzheimer's as we feel there is nothing to gain for any of us from her knowing.

7th April – Canterbury

Bought and read the local paper today as it contained the article Gerry wrote following his visit a few days ago. The headline of the article reads: 'Former head takes lead in fight against Alzheimer's'. In the article Gerry includes accurate facts from the Alzheimer's Society website, and then a piece about me outlining how outwardly I appear to be little changed from the last time he saw me, but also referring to the hammer blow that the diagnosis and the disease was causing me, and other people with it who also have Alzheimer's disease.

The article outlines a few of my activities that I'm doing in London and Kent on behalf of KMPT. He also covers activities that I'm doing outside of dementia, both with my family, and going into Wincheap School to hear readers, alongside the continuation of my interest in hobbies. The photographs were from my final assembly at Blean, and a really good one of Ian, Reinhard and me at the Alzheimer's Disease International conference.

10th April – Canterbury

Jo Pullen from the SILK (Social Inclusion Living in Kent) project has asked my thoughts about a book that they're producing called *The Dementia Diaries*. It's a unique book written by four or five teenagers with a professional writer (Matthew Snyman). I think it's largely based on personal experience of grandparents within their family and is in the style of *Diary of a Wimpy Kid* (by Jeff Kinney) which many of the children at Wincheap seem to be currently reading. It was illuminating to read about dementia through the eyes of youngsters. It should be a really good book when it's eventually available. Also, Jo spoke to me about an embryonic idea they've got to establish buddies for people who have been recently diagnosed with dementia. She wants my thoughts on whether I could be involved in advising, or actually being a buddy.

13th April – Canterbury

After considering this since the ADI conference, we had the first official meeting at St Martin's Hospital to discuss an activist role which Reinhard and the Trust are keen to establish. At the meeting were myself, Reinhard, Janet Lloyd from the Trust, and Ian, the student supporter.

It was a very positive meeting. I prepared beforehand what I thought was a draft job description, and this was easily agreed. The hardest part was thinking of a title for the role. At the end of the day, we have settled upon the title 'KMPT dementia activist'.

15th April – Canterbury

I've been thinking a lot about the meeting I had two days ago at St Martin's about the role that I am taking on. I had decided that 'champion' was too high a bar to set. The label of 'ambassador' has been taken by the Alzheimer's Society, 'advocate' has legal implications, and Dr Nick Branch, my son-in-law, thought that the word 'activist' conjures up ideas of someone being in confrontation with the NHS and associated professionals who I am wishing to work with, who had just come from the barricades wearing a balaclava! Nick and I have put our heads together, and he has come up with the role title 'envoy', which I emailed to Reinhard and Janet today. They're absolutely delighted to hear this, and are both very happy to support the title. So as from today, 15th April 2012, I will now carry to meetings and conferences the label of Kent and Medway Dementia Service user envoy.

Reflecting also today on how I've been. Sometimes I feel better, but I seldom feel well.

17th April – Canterbury

With my new label (but no badge yet!) I attended today a consultation road show, organised by the East Kent NHS Trust, examining beds and wards at St Martin's Hospital and beyond. Barbara Beats, my consultant, was one of the speakers on the platform, and I met and had a conversation with Justine Leonard, who is one of the senior managers at the Trust. I had previously met Justine when I spoke to the Trust board with Reinhard, and knowing the importance of networking I sense she is a positive ally for the cause of service user involvement we are seeking to advance.

26th April – Canterbury

Another meeting with Jo from SILK, Tom, a carer, and Ian, supporting me to discuss the Buddies idea. As there are only two of us it's clearly going to need more people to come along if this idea is going to work. I'm not happy in taking on this role in the isolation that I sense around it at the moment.

28th April – Canterbury

A bright, sunny spring day and the regular meeting with Reinhard today took place outside on my patio. Amongst the topics we discussed was a concern Reinhard had clearly been sitting on. After the conference on 12th March, Ian apparently spoke to Reinhard around a comment made to him from one of the audience, who said how concerned he was about people like me doing this activist work, and how one is able to cope when it comes to a close because of the disease. He had fears for my health over this and, indeed, mentioned suicide. Ian was worried by this and didn't know what to do with this information, so confided in Reinhard, who then spoke to me about it. I was quite surprised by this, and stressed to Reinhard that there were no concerns on that front at all, and to please pass this on to Ian, but not to share it with Rosemary for fear of upsetting her.

30th April – Canterbury

Today I was interviewing at St Martin's Hospital. It's my first NHS-related interview, and the first I've been involved in since I retired. A community nurse post based at St Martin's for the Home Treatment team is available. I think it is an early example by KMPT of involving service users, because I got no sense that this was something they've done before. Celia, another person with dementia who shared the responsibility with me, felt positive about the day. Both Celia and I are ex-teachers and have interviewed in the past professionally. One interviewee was rather better than the other, although we didn't conclude at the end who was going to get the job. The professionals present have assured us that they will inform us.

16th May – Canterbury

Now I'm retired, Rosemary and I have more time to attend the cinema. Often we do this is on Wednesday morning for a programme of films called the 'Senior Screen'. This week, the film was *The Artist*, which has attracted a lot of publicity and been awarded a number of Oscars. It's a silent film set in the 1920s. I found it incredibly boring, in fact I would describe it as one of the worst films I remember seeing.

Thinking of the word 'artist', I find writing a journal and my diary as being a bit like doing a painting. Rosemary's a very able amateur artist, and I know how much care and thought she puts into her artwork, how she lays down a wash, and then builds the picture up gradually as it begins to take shape. My journals which supplement my diary with reflections on the key days are a bit like that, the wash being scribbled notes, and coherent sentences coming later as I seek to make thoughts more comprehensible. I am unsure how I will use my journal or what I will use it for, or whose eyes will see it beyond mine.

25th May – Maidstone

I was keen to attend my first Young Onset Dementia Network meeting at Maidstone with Reinhard and Ian. I really enjoyed this meeting. I feel well when I am treated with trust and respect, and regarded as a part of a small professional mental health team, enabling me to view those around the table as colleagues, and to be treated in the same way. I was asked by Reinhard to give a short presentation to the group around person-centred approaches, and something around the impacts and coping strategies connected to dementia, how I deal with them, and how professionals can help us with dementia's impacts.

To conclude my presentation, I explained my envoy role, so that those around the table were aware at least of my existence and what I'm able to bring to the role and to the Trust.

26th May – Faversham

Today we had our annual EKIDS group visit. This year it was to Shepherd Neame's brewery in Faversham. Needless to say, this event was very well supported by the group with a really good turnout. We had an excellent tour of the brewery, and the opportunity to try a little sample, and then buy some of the wares at the end. Whilst recently I have read some research about the possible benefits of a glass of red wine for those with dementia, I am unaware of potential gains connected to beer, but what I do know is that today was a very friendly and harmonious one and that to see inside a brewery for the first time was as enjoyable as tasting the final product – in moderation of course!

28th May – Canterbury

At the hospital for my six-monthly appointment with Dr Beats to catch up with her. Within 10 or 15 minutes, I was able to update her on how up and down I've been lately, though still remaining positive. I did outline to her something about my sense of decline cognitively, but emotionally and psychologically I feel good most of the time. I was able to talk to her a little about my activities in the envoy role, and that I do something related to the role once every week or two. We discussed my diet, and the fact that I'm still okay on the medication.

I asked her about a care plan, but still nothing of what I would describe as useful is forthcoming, although she did promise me that she would refer me back to the memory clinic so that Elizabeth Field and Jouko could possibly do a two-year update check on me, and then report back to her, which in turn will be conveyed to me.

30th May – London

After my generally positive initial experience of the DAA (Dementia Action Alliance) today, it was off to a quarterly meeting in London with Reinhard and Ian. The DAA appears to be an organisation that I can readily relate to and become involved with. My place in the DAA is supported by Dementia UK, who technically support carers, but because of some of the work I've done with them, they're very happy to sponsor my involvement. It was the first time I met Sarah Tilsed and Simon Kitchen, who lead and coordinate the DAA.

When I got home from the meeting, there was a very supportive letter from the local NHS, connected to my application for a bus pass. I'll forward that now to Kent County Council, and as I am deemed disabled I can hopefully secure the bus pass, which will help me to remain both independent and interdependent.

1st June – Canterbury

As part of my involvement in going to hear children read at Wincheap School they invited me along today to enjoy their Queen's Jubilee Party. It was a really pleasant event. The sun shone, and there were lots of happy children and parents there, some of whom I recognised. It was also clear that the teachers were very relaxed and engaged.

A letter arrived from Elizabeth Field about the request from Dr Beats for a retest. Elizabeth has been able to offer me an appointment, which she says could take two hours on 11th October – good, but four months away!

6th June – Canterbury

Whilst in the garden, Rosemary fortuitously went out the front to do something, and who should be arriving on our drive, unbeknown to us, but

Garry Golder, the Australian teacher who I had done the job and house exchange with in 1989.

Seeing him, you could have knocked us both down with a feather. I hadn't seen Garry for some years, nor had any contact from him. He and his wife were on holiday in the UK and staying with friends in Canterbury. We chatted for about 30 minutes in the garden. He didn't want to come inside or have a cup of tea, but we stood in the sunshine amiably chatting. He was interested to know how I was, because he had heard through the grapevine that I had been unwell, and that I was now living with Alzheimer's. Rosemary and I were both impressed by his thoughtfulness in coming to see us.

19th June – Canterbury

Enjoyed a really good dementia workshop at Canterbury Christ Church University, led by Professor Jan Dewing and Professor Brendan McCormick. One of the key activities at the event was craft focused. All the other participants were professionals and chose to draw the image of dementia through an A3-sized pictorial image, whereas I chose a template of a mask. The mask for me is important, because at times I feel I wear a mask, although not in reality. The mask I constructed had lots of bright colour as I like wearing bright colours after years of drab business attire. It also had tears coming down my cheeks but with lines through the tears. At times I feel psychologically battered, so I drew a small bruise on the chin. Brendan seemed interested in my mask and asked me to explain it to the group, which I was happy to do.

21st June – Canterbury

Gaynor Smith, the service user involvement manager from the Alzheimer's Society, visited me. I met Gaynor at Canterbury East station, and we walked in the sunshine along the Stour Way. I think she was quite surprised that we took this route. Although impressed, I don't think she quite knew what to make of it, but I thought it showed her something about the area where we live. We talked whilst we walked, alongside the river and marshes, and when we got to my home we discussed in greater depth training for Alzheimer's Society staff, which we could work on together. We then moved on to talk about the new dementia guide that the society are looking to produce as a book to give out to people at point of diagnosis.

At around about this point, we were joined by a professional photographer who wanted to take pictures of me in our garden, which will apparently be used to promote the new guide.

30th June–9th July – St Austell, Cornwall

Rosemary and I had our summer holiday in Cornwall again this year. Whilst the weather wasn't very good, one of the highlights for us was a visit to the Eden Project, which we found absolutely fascinating and fortunately it did remain dry that day. Also, we took in the Maritime Museum in Falmouth, which we also found interesting. The comfortable bed and breakfast we stayed in was in the pleasant village of Polgooth. As I felt well during the week I did not feel the need to tell anyone that I had dementia.

11th July – Folkestone

Today I attended a post-diagnostic group called Living Well with Dementia with Elizabeth Field in Folkestone at the Broadmeadow centre. My role within this presentation was to inform the group of newly diagnosed people with young onset dementia that it is possible to live well after the diagnosis, and I gave them a number of suggestions about coping with dementia, largely around the area of remaining physically and mentally active. I was able to signpost them towards what support was available, and to encourage them to access some of that support. Alongside this I feel strongly that people should establish their lasting power of attorney and wills while they still have the mental capacity to do so, and I used mine and Rosemary's example of setting it up soon after diagnosis and then parking it until it's required.

15th July – Ramsgate

We enjoyed an afternoon strawberry tea today, organised by the EKIDS group, and funded by me from a donation I was given from the interviewing at St Martin's. I still don't know who got the job! I don't feel it appropriate to keep the money, and I want to ensure that it goes to something useful, hence the idea of providing all 20 of us with an afternoon strawberry tea. It was great fun.

17th July – Canterbury

Rosemary and I joined a group of people from Canterbury Christ Church University in the Dane John Gardens for a picnic, which was to mark the sad departure of Penny Hibberd from the dementia centre at the university. Penny has been a good ally, and a good friend over the past year or so, and has opened a number of doors to me alongside encouraging me in the roles that I have taken on. She will be missed, both by myself and, more importantly, by the centre at the university. But it's interesting around the notion of one door opening, and one door closing, because at the picnic, I met and had a long conversation with Pat Chung, who is the head of occupational therapy (OT) at the university, and we plan to work collaboratively in the future.

19th July – Canterbury

The Olympic torch visited Canterbury, and Rosemary and I walked into Wincheap to watch the athletes run along the main street. This will be the closest we'll get to involvement in the Olympics, because when the lottery was announced for tickets, I wasn't sure how well I would be by 2012, so I didn't consider applying for tickets for any events. I now recognise that I am well enough to attend, and would have been able to, but I didn't know that 18 months ago when I envisaged my decline being more rapid than in fact it has been.

Having joined the crowds to watch the Olympic torch be carried through Canterbury has given us some sense of attachment to the event.

21st July – Canterbury

The sun shone down on us today for an interesting walk with the University of the Third Age, around the St Martin's area of Canterbury, including a visit to St Augustine's Abbey. The leader of the group was Martin. St Augustine's Abbey has historic connections generally, but also to me, because in the 1980s, when I was a young teacher working at Pilgrim's Way School, my class and I worked on a publication for schools using the abbey, which was funded by English Heritage. I still have a copy of the book, and am pleased to know it's still used by schools that visit the site.

24th July – London

First visit to the Alzheimer's Society headquarters at Devon House, near St Katharine Docks. This was to attend a service user involvement group with Rosemary. When we arrived at Victoria Station there was a lot of razzmatazz about the forthcoming Olympics. We took the underground to

Tower Hill and then the short walk to St Katharine Docks, sidetracking to take a peep at Tower Bridge, which had the Olympic rings festooned upon it. Impressive.

At the Devon House meeting I was introduced to a small number of other service users, including two names which stuck with me. One was former GP Dr Jennifer Bute, and the other was Larry Gardiner, who is about my age, comes from Oxford, and has young onset dementia but clearly is still keen to be involved and to be an advocate and activist.

25th July – Lullingstone

Our annual outing with the Wednesday Club from Shepherdswell this year was to Lullingstone Castle in northwest Kent to see their World Garden. This was a site Rosemary and I had visited a couple of years ago with her sister Barbara and her husband Michael. The garden and the castle are run by a gentleman called Tom Hart Dyke, who is related to Miranda Hart. He is famous for having been kidnapped a few years ago in Colombia when he was plant gathering, and has since written a book about his adventures. This led to the creation of a world garden, where each continent's plants are represented within a very impressive and beautiful garden.

9th August – Canterbury

Recently Kent County Council asked me to speak at ten events over a two-week period across the county to help train their staff in dementia, including staff who work in the libraries, the museums, the art galleries and in the Gateway Services. I said I simply couldn't do this, so the council found some money to commission Dementia UK to make a film of me speaking in my home environment. This will now be used at the venues which I'm not able to attend. Today was the day when we did the filming.

The film was made by a professional film maker working for Dementia UK named Mycal Miller. Mycal filmed me in the lounge talking about dementia and in the garden, and then filmed Rosemary and me near where we live with footage by the river, and walking alongside the Hambrook Marshes. Mycal was very sensitive and considerate to our needs, as well as being very well prepared and supportive.

He mentioned about possibly putting the film into a more public place later, but I'm not sure who would want to watch it.

16th August – Tunbridge Wells

Still in filming mode, this time at the Salomons Centre at Canterbury Christ Church University. Laura and Helen, who are responsible for coordinating the psychology doctorate course at the Salomons Centre, had recently met me at my home. They wanted me to speak to students on the course, but Salomons isn't an easy place for me to get to, so the idea was that Rosemary would take me there today, and the university would film me talking about various aspects of dementia, which they could then use with the students. I made copious notes, which I took with me, around how and why I wish to be involved with the doctorate course. I explained through the film how important it was to see the person and not just the symptoms and, moving on from that, to recognise the importance of service user involvement in psychological services, and in dementia care generally. I outlined the process of my diagnosis, and the importance of clinical psychology.

Next, I moved on to talking about coping strategies, and how I do my best to live well and remain positive despite what the disease throws at me. The importance of research was covered, when I talked about user involvement within research. Finally, I concluded that whilst I do feel somewhat 'bulletproof' at the moment, I recognise that two years after diagnosis Alzheimer's is having an impact upon me.

18th August – Whitstable

At the Strode Gallery in Whitstable Rosemary concluded a two-week art exhibition with others from her art class. The quality of Rosemary's artwork is superb, as indeed is that of many of the other artists within the group. She was delighted to have sold two paintings and a number of cards she had made from her paintings.

19th–21st August – Nottingham

We visited Nottingham in order to celebrate and mark my mother's 80th birthday with her in the care home. The care home made a special cake for her, which she enjoyed, because my mother is always partial to a bit of cake!

28th August – Canterbury

Met with Pat Chung following up our picnic conversation a few weeks ago to discuss working with her, and how she may be able to engage me within the occupational therapy course at the university as a guest lecturer. I enjoyed talking to Pat about dementia, OT and also our common interest in Hong Kong. I'm really looking forward to developing this project.

30th August – Canterbury

Julia Burton-Jones from Dementia UK visited me at home to discuss the NICE (National Institute for Health and Care Excellence) guidelines on dementia. Julia has been commissioned to seek the views of service users on the guidelines, and she thinks that I am well placed to advise on this. I am realising the potential of these exercises, but also their limitations, and am mindful of the need for the views of those with lived experience to be genuinely involved, as is the case with Julia, rather than considered as tokenistic gestures.

6th September – Canterbury

A periodic meeting at St Martin's Hospital entitled the KMPT Service User Forum. There were a range of local organisations, including Age UK, present, and we talked about how services in the region can be better devised and targeted to meet the needs of older adults, including those with dementia. At my age and stage of dementia I am not sure how representative I am of those who are being discussed.

7th September – Canterbury

Back at St Martin's today to meet the new students with Reinhard. There are two female students this year building upon Ian's experience, Heather and Emily, both of whom seem very pleasant, and quite eager to learn. However, I sense a feeling of apprehension and a sense of how difficult it will be to follow in the footsteps of Ian, who has returned to university to complete his degree.

8th–15th September – Jersey

This is my first visit to the island since I holidayed there as an 11-year-old child in 1967. Rosemary and I flew from Manston to Jersey Airport, which was great, because Manston Airport is a small airport just outside Ramsgate, and the check-in was so easy, taking about an hour. The car park is a five-minute walk from the terminal, and the plane a two-minute stroll from the terminal. All very small, all very easy to navigate and to manage.

After a smooth flight we had a relaxing, comfortable holiday during which the sun shone most of the week. We saw much of what the island provides by hiring a little Ford Fiesta, which served our purposes during the week. Highlights visited included Portelet Bay, St Brelade's Bay and Gorey, and the only day when it rained, Rosemary and I went to visit the German underground hospital created by slave labour during World War II. It brought back memories for me of going there with my parents the last time I was on the island.

19th September – Ashford

I gave a talk with Mycal Miller and county librarian Tricia Fincher to approximately 30 Kent County Council library and Gateway staff. I'm reminded of a quote from Isak Dinesen, who said, 'To be a person is to have a story to tell,' and today I tried to fulfil that by telling my story with Mycal's help. What he did was plant me in the audience when we were doing the opening activities. One of these was for everybody to write down something from their past, something from their present, and something from their future. The idea was to illustrate that people with dementia have a past, arguably a present, but very few would consider them to have much of a future. He discussed that with the participants.

As I no longer work for Kent County Council I sensed people wondering why I was there, and at this point Mycal called me to the front. He introduced me as someone whose mother had Alzheimer's, and I recognised people accepting that that's why I was attending. He then conducted a question and answer session with me, asking about my experience of my mother having dementia, and how that had impacted upon me, alongside how her disease had progressed to this point. Then he showed the film that he'd made with me recently. I'd seen the film before, so I spent my time watching the audience. Their faces were a picture. They were amazed. The guy sitting in front of them who had just previously been talking about his mother was now there, unfolding in front of their eyes, disclosing that he too has Alzheimer's. You could have heard a pin drop. You could have felt the air being sucked out of the room. Everyone was stunned. Although invited to do so, no one asked a question, and we followed this with a break during which no one came forward to speak to me. They seemed almost in shock and disbelief and coped by keeping their distance, which made me feel uncomfortable.

25th September – London

Attended the Dementia Action Alliance quarterly meeting in London with Reinhard and Heather, the student. I feel fully behind the aims of the Dementia Action Alliance as it seeks to unite professionals and people affected by dementia in making the world a more dementia-friendly place, alongside improving services for those with dementia, and raising the knowledge level of professionals working in dementia care.

In addition, it has a number of calls to action. At the moment, they are focusing on dementia-friendly communities, and there was a really good presentation by Trevor Jarvis, a man with dementia, and Graham Whippy, who works for Lloyds Bank. It's really interesting to see that Lloyds are promoting dementia-friendly banking: food for thought for anyone with dementia considering changing their bank. There was also a call to action for carers from a strong carer presence, or rather, a very strong former carer presence. I looked at the other people who were advocates or activists there, people like Peter Ashley, Trevor Jarvis, Peter Dunlop. I watched and listened to them speak. I remained quiet, and tried to take in what I was listening to. I tried to think about the experience, and to learn from these people.

2nd October – Whitstable

Mycal Miller and I repeated the same event we had done at Ashford recently. These are the two of the ten events that I can possibly do, working with Kent frontline service staff. We used exactly the same format and it worked precisely the same way as it did on 19th September with the same impact, although this time I was pleased that people did speak to me at the break.

5th October – Canterbury

Following on from the meetings and conversations I've had with Pat Chung, today was an opportunity for me to begin working with her by delivering a talk to third-year undergraduate occupational therapy students at Canterbury Christ Church University. She gave me the luxury of speaking for two hours, and I filled that time. I spoke to the students about why it's important to support the training of occupational therapists. As with all my talks, it was written specifically with this audience in mind.

The talk needed to be useful to the students on the course. I utilised music because I had the time to do so, and I played them songs from my playlist: Labi Siffre's 'Something Inside So Strong', 'Won't Give In', by Sara Storer, and 'While I Am Here', by Eric Bogle. All those three songs mean a lot to me as they describe how I try and live my life.

My talk then outlined the symptoms of dementia, and broadened their understanding, which really was, at the beginning, solely that dementia affects the memory of the elderly. They had no idea about the diagnosis process, which I explained to them alongside what coping strategies I employ, and how occupational therapy can support people. I explained how I feel physically, emotionally and psychologically, and what negative triggers bring down the fog. They were interested to know also about the impact that my Alzheimer's has on those closest to me, such as my wife and my family.

Finally, I concluded by explaining to them my role as an envoy and what I'm trying to do to help raise awareness.

11th October – Canterbury

Today was the appointment at St Martin's Hospital I was given four months ago by Elizabeth Field, to meet with her and Jouko again to conduct a series of tests two years after my initial assessment by them. I talked through my concerns, as they gave me an opportunity and a platform to do so, and, alongside that, I talked about my positive approach. I used the weather analogy of 'foggy and sunny days'.

The assessment included reading a story which I had to recount, and I felt I did fine with that. I then was asked to read some print and tell them some words beginning with the letter 'D' or 'R' or 'C'. I had to track some letters, which I found very hard, and some numbers, which I found easier. They then gave me a series of shapes to copy. I don't know how well I did overall. I'm meeting with Elizabeth and Jouko in two weeks' time to get the results.

25th October – Canterbury

Back at the hospital with Rosemary for the appointment with Elizabeth to get the results of the tests. She began by saying that the results were pretty much as expected two years after a diagnosis of dementia. She explained the wider context of activities to both of us, including the impact that has on both myself and Rosemary. It is always useful to be reminded of this. She said that there had been a slight decline in my memory, but that my executive function, generally speaking, remained very similar. One of the tests that she used with me was called RBANS, where there had been a slight decline in most areas. For the list of words and the story, my ability had declined by 20 per cent. My competence in using numbers and alphabetical order had also declined, the latter more noticeably so.

Coming away in the car, having explained this to Rosemary, in the moments of silence I was reminded of a Chinese proverb which goes something like 'Eat bitter to taste sweet', i.e. you go through difficult times to enjoy a brighter future. I really sense this at the moment. These are difficult times, but I'm trying to restore my former drive in order to achieve a brighter future. Though what that future entails, I don't know.

30th October – Maidstone

Today Reinhard took me to Maidstone to attend a conference with the NHS, and from this onto Brighton for the UK Dementia Congress (UKDC). Ian and Rosemary are going straight from Canterbury to Brighton and we'll meet them there. The conference in Maidstone had a really full agenda, and was very comprehensive in what it was trying to achieve. There was a strong presence from the NHS in Kent, the Alzheimer's Society and other charities. There must have been 80 to 90 people in the audience, amongst whom I met Tanya, who presented on dementia care mapping. I was impressed by Tanya's approach and I hope to be able to meet up with her in future and to do work together since she's based in East Kent.

I was though alarmed by a couple of things during the day. In the entrance hall, some of the posters projecting the image of dementia, used by the Alzheimer's Society, were really very startling, sobering and depressing. Also, I shared the platform with Julie, a carer, whose husband, Bob, had not long before been diagnosed with young onset dementia. He appears to be more progressed into the disease than I am. A couple of things stuck with me. First, she said that, at the diagnosis, she went in a wife and came out a carer. That shook me for starters. Then following on from his diagnosis, she used the image of post-diagnostic support as being a magical mystery tour, that she hadn't got a clue where to go and what was available. Not a good picture, but many would say an accurate one.

In my 25-minute slot, I tried to seek a balance between reality and positivity. I started by explaining the person who I am, and I really laboured the point to the audience today because I thought it appropriate. I talked about diagnosis, and the immediate period after diagnosis, likening it to a cliff-edge moment, which was consistent with Julie's talk.

I then explored how the situation could be improved for others: how staff development and training should be improved in order that those working with us are more aware of the needs of people with dementia. I talked about GPs and the important role they play, and how often they can be obstructive rather than constructive, although with me that wasn't the case.

I talked to the audience about care plans, and how we need one at the point of diagnosis, not at point of entry into a care home or a crisis. We need better, and more, post-diagnostic services, using my phrase 'spend one pound to save two'. I think that message got through to the audience. There's a greater need for more awareness, more people coming forward to speak, better communication between us, and understanding the person, as well as the dementia.

31st October – Brighton

Rosemary, Reinhard, Ian and I attended our first UK Dementia Congress together with our poster and a talk. The poster is the same as the one we used at ADI, and the talk was entitled 'Developing the role of envoy in Kent'. Although slotted into the conference agenda at 8.30 a.m., I enjoyed our talk very much alongside Ian and Reinhard. A real privilege. I began by listening to Ian and Reinhard, who gave the background. They talked about Kitwood, before moving on to dementia activists Christine Bryden, Richard Taylor and Kate Swaffer. All of whom live abroad. Who are our British role models?

Next, they moved on to talking about how the Department of Health, since 2001, has been trying to entrench and develop service user involvement. From small acorns big trees grow, but as we know this takes time. Then Ian and I outlined the project we had constructed together, the use of the pro formas, and the psychological analysis of the data he did.

The important part for me was to speak to the audience about my aims for the role around confronting prejudice and stigma, providing a useful service user perspective to professionals within the NHS and the voluntary sector, to raise the profile of people with dementia, to allow professionals to better understand how it is possible to live well with dementia, and then to apply that to those who have the disease. I see my role as being that of a critical professional friend to service providers.

There was a recognition of the increased demand on my time and energy, for which I need support. The talk was well received by the audience, and I got the sense that they'd not heard something like this before.

4th November – Canterbury

Received a telephone call from a script writer named James Coleman, who's writing a script for a BBC drama on young onset dementia. He'd been given my name by Dementia UK. He asked me questions around what it is like to live with dementia, aged mid-50s, and I was able to tell him from the inside what it was really like. James promised to keep me informed about the project which, realistically, he said could take years to bring to the screen.

6th November – Canterbury

Jo from the Alzheimer's Society press team ran a telephone interview with me about David Cameron's launch of the Prime Minister's 'challenge on dementia' in 2012. They wanted some quotes and some thoughts from me on this crucially important initiative. This was my first real contact from the society's press team, and I hope that it's the first of many.

11th November – Canterbury

Brett, one of Reinhard's colleagues from West Kent, asked me to help him prepare a document for KMPT in order to try to improve the diagnosis rates in the county, which are below the national average; the national average is 42 per cent, and Kent and Medway's rate trails behind at 38 per cent. My view is that both the low figure and the comparison are deeply disturbing. Brett was very open to, and appreciative of, my comments.

16th November – Canterbury

Potentially an important day – the first network meeting for service users. We met at the Thanington Resource Centre to launch the group. There were two students, two psychologists (Reinhard and Elizabeth), and five people with dementia – four men, and one woman.

We were also joined by Nick Dent from KMPT, who told us that something like this had been done before. I didn't agree, because I see this group as being innovative and unique for this area. What he had in mind was quite different, and I used with him the metaphor of a bakery, where we don't want biscuits, we don't want cake, not even if cream cake – we want to share the keys to the bakery!

I think that had quite an impact upon him, not necessarily a positive one. But the point was that we would be in joint control with the professionals leading this group, and not dictated to by the Trust.

The context for this group is that the diagnosis rate for dementia in Kent is below the national average, which in itself is extremely low, and its provision of after-diagnosis care is also really poor. There's very little service user involvement in the dementia field, beyond small projects which are useful for those involved, but have no direct bearing upon policy and upon the care given to others in the county. This is a watershed moment, I feel. The group is seeking to raise awareness, not just for us, but with us, and links very much to the Prime Minister's challenge around professionals and service users working together. We are seeking change and improvements. We are looking to help make things better. It's going to be hard, we know, but as a group of professionals and people with a diagnosis there is a lot more we can achieve. Now established, we agree we will meet at the same venue on the second Friday of every month. Whilst the group has no name yet, we have lots of enthusiasm, and that is a good way to start.

20th November – Canterbury

We both attended Age UK Canterbury for a computer lesson, partly to improve Rosemary and my computer skills, but also to show loyalty to Age UK who have been incredibly supportive to us, and had signposted us to this as something which they thought we might find useful.

22nd November – London

The DAA annual meeting attended with Reinhard. This was at the Central Hall, Westminster, and the highlight for me was Dawn Brooker, who spoke within a debate against the motion that the NHS is Europe's leader in dementia care. Reinhard reminded me that I'd met Dawn at the ADI, back in March. She spoke very eloquently with a degree of humour and consequently got my vote.

Jeremy Hunt, the newly appointed minister of state, also spoke. Last year it was Andrew Lansley, who I didn't rate very highly. Jeremy Hunt, although some of his policies suggest otherwise, did speak with some compassion and conviction about his role, and about what he is seeking to achieve for those with dementia who are utilising NHS services.

I was also made aware of the Care Quality Commission (CQC), and their director Philip King gave a very eloquent, interesting speech.

I was sponsored for the event by Dementia UK, but actually from now on, I'm going to be listed as an affiliate of the DAA.

On the way home, Reinhard had another event, so he took me as far as St Pancras, and then we separated in a café. I don't know St Pancras very well, and I got lost and asked a policeman the way.

26th November – Canterbury

I saw my consultant, Dr Beats, at Kent and Canterbury Hospital. She went through my medication and asked me how things were going. She also talked through what Elizabeth Field and Jouko had completed with me by way of the two-year assessment, but didn't give me any kind of care plan beyond checking that the medication was not harming me, and was possibly doing some good. She ended by setting the next appointment for six months' time.

6th December – Whitstable

The library service have been very supportive through their interest in my story, and in utilising me to talk to staff. Today, however, they asked me to deliver a talk to the public, which I did at Swalecliffe Library very close to where I was a deputy head in the 1990s. I guess 15 people turned up, mostly people around the age of 60 to 70. I spoke about having dementia, which surprised them, because they had never met anyone who was my age with dementia. Also, I talked about how I felt, both the positives and the negatives, linking this to triggers and coping strategies, and ended with a lot of time discussing the stereotypical image of those with dementia. One bonus for me from the morning was that David Smith, my old boss from Swalecliffe, called in at the end of the talk to see how I was.

13th December – London

I travelled on the high-speed train with Rosemary to a meeting at Devon House, to review the Alzheimer's Society service user involvement plan.

Larry Gardiner, who I'd met before at a service user involvement group, was there, and he spoke eloquently, knowledgeably and passionately about the society's role in engaging with and involving people with dementia.

14th December – Canterbury

Met with Heather, a placement student, largely to discuss her project, which she's doing on the dementia service user network. We still haven't got a name for the group, so at the moment it's called the Dementia Service User Network. Heather seemed quite distressed about aspects of her placement which she wanted to share with me. I listened and advised her primarily to speak to those involved in her professional network. She left happier than she arrived.

17th December – Canterbury

I always feel that Christmas really begins at the point where primary schools perform their Christmas Nativity plays. I used to love sitting in Blean school hall watching the children when I was head, and also attending the Nativity plays of our own children when they were at primary school. I hadn't been to one now for two or three years, since I retired, so to have the opportunity to go into Wincheap to watch theirs was a rare treat.

I do enjoy going into Wincheap to hear the children read, and whilst the staff wax lyrical about what I bring to it, I feel I take as much, if not more, from the time spent there, sharing the enthusiasm and the engagement of the children, and the fact that I enjoy feeling part of a team, as I'm made most welcome by the staff.

19th December – Ashford

I co-presented today with Tanya at a dementia excellence event in Ashford. This was for champions working in care homes, and utilised Tanya's expertise in dementia care matters. She wanted to film me telling my life story, and to show the film at the event. We did it in the same way as I did with Mycal, introducing me initially as someone whose mother had Alzheimer's, and again it worked perfectly with this audience.

Alongside the usual elements of my talks, which are around the impact of dementia and coping strategies, again, written with the specific audience in mind, in this case care home staff, I went on to explore what I hope for when I move to a care home at some point in the future. We stressed the importance of the work of Kitwood and Dawn Brooker linked to ensuring that I'm valued; I'm treated as an individual; my life history is incorporated into my care; I'm shown empathy, through relationships built and nurtured by interactions with staff and other residents; and that I'm stimulated by both the environment and those that I'm with, supported by staff who are well trained and motivated.

I then outlined my thoughts about the environment in the care home, ending with a lengthy discussion about what challenging behaviour means, then steering the care home staff to thinking about behaviour brought about by frustration.

23rd–27th December – Canterbury and Thanet

The family gathered for Christmas activities, including our annual Christmas Day picnic on the beach irrespective of the weather with champagne and savoury snacks.

31st December – Canterbury

No celebrating for New Year again. Looking back at 2012, and forward to 2013, I'm reminded of a book I was reading recently, which had a quote from the gravestone of Yorkshire novelist Winifred Holtby: 'God give me work, till my life shall end, and life to my work till my work is done.' That is often how I see my life.

Sometime in 2012

Dear Alzheimer's

The past year has flown by, and the busier I become the more able I feel to keep your creeping presence at bay. Some days I'm extra tired but I overcome this and am keeping well despite your efforts to sabotage this.

To keep you at bay, one strategy you will have noticed is that I have adopted my long-held professional philosophy that information is power. Perhaps you smugly see yourself as the expert? To counter the imbalance that you benefit from, in being seen as the expert and I the learner, I am reading all I can about dementia from both the professional perspective and those living with you. I know this is not enough, which is why I attend meetings and conferences so that my armoury against you can continue to be effective.

I know I offended and challenged you in my last letter by outlining that I have a growing network of allies who stand alongside me, and I recognise at times that you try to infiltrate this network. Now that I am viewed by professional friends and colleagues as an envoy, this will provide me with extra tools in my toolkit to outwit you and tip the scales more in my favour.

You have in the past attempted to influence the media and encourage them to portray your victories. Recently though they have been exposed to the newly launched Prime Minister's challenge on dementia. You see, even our country's leader is lined up in opposition to you and will bring enormous resources to bear in the effort to get the better of you.

In addition to my human allies I now have another in the form of medication: galantamine. You know my aversion to pharmacological treatments, but taking a tablet produced from the sap of daffodils grown at altitude in the Welsh hills fills me with pleasure. After cold, dark winter days the daffodil not only heralds spring, but resistance to your cold clutches. For too long there have been no new drugs to defeat your evil approaches, but there is light at the end of the tunnel. Now a growing desire by the Alzheimer's Society, Alzheimer's Research UK and others to invest more in research will stop you in your tracks. This will protect other people you may identify as targets for you to reside within in future. I have joined the Research Network and rest assured I will do EVERYTHING I can to help to defeat you.

I remain, resoundingly positively

Keith

2013

—

'Building a role'

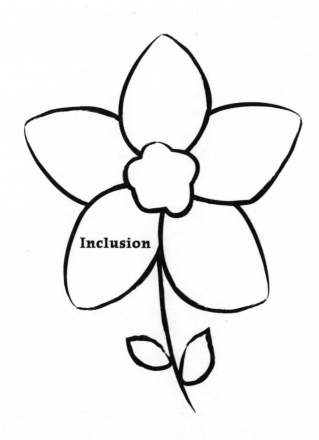

Inclusion

11th January – Canterbury

For some while I have been considering doing something completely different which might stimulate my brain and give me a different outlet – one which would serve my creative and intellectual needs, be interesting and draw me away from becoming too dementia focused, and avoid the risk of becoming a 'one-trick pony'. Today gave me the opportunity to make a start by beginning a life writing course at Canterbury Christ Church University. The course tutor is April Doyle, and my hope is that I will have the confidence to take on the challenge of life writing.

Recently I've been feeling extra tired on these long, dark nights and short, cold winter days which seem to sap my energy more than usual. Despite this, at the start of the new year, I've decided to ban four words from my vocabulary: 'can't', 'sufferer', 'but' and 'regret'.

In the case of 'can't', this links into my understanding of Kitwood and focusing on what *can* be done.

I now hate the word 'sufferer', despite the fact that reading through my diary two years ago, I was using it to describe myself to professionals. I worry about the fact that people would regard me as a sufferer and then define and treat me as such.

The small word 'but' has a huge significance. It negates whatever went before. It's so easy to say, 'I would help you but – I'm too busy.'

'Regret', often brought on by dwelling on what one might have done or could have done, is not helpful. I've always tried not to have regrets, and now I am going to try and ban it from my vocabulary and thinking.

12th January – Canterbury

Rosemary and I went to the cinema to see *Les Misérables*. I was immensely impressed and moved by the story. Although vastly different, the film stirred my emotions and transported me back to a time when I was a student in the 1970s, marching in London and demonstrating in Sheffield as part of the campaign against education cuts. At that time, I sensed a real feeling that we could change the world through comradeship, which in turn reinforced many of my friendships with fellow students.

15th January – Dartford

Reinhard and I attended a young onset dementia meeting as part of the KMPT efforts to improve professional knowledge around living with young onset dementia. Ian came with us, and at the event I met David Prothero, a former carer. David spoke eloquently about his wife, who was an ex-teacher and had young onset dementia.

I took the opportunity to speak with Trust staff about young onset. I'm now gaining more confidence in presenting alongside Reinhard. The subject of my talk was a positive approach to coping. Alongside me on stage were Ian and Reinhard, talking about our service user involvement project from 2011 to 2012.

17th January – Tunbridge Wells

Canterbury Christ Church University Salomons Centre is not easy to reach from Canterbury as it is set in the heart of the Kent Weald outside Tunbridge Wells. Reinhard drove, and it was a delight to meet his line manager, Alison Culverwell, for the first time. The event was to launch the South East England Dementia Centre. The conference had some positive aspects, not least of which was networking. It was good to meet Jan Dewing, who's taken over from Penny Hibberd in running the dementia centre.

20th January – Canterbury

Heavy snowfall today. Eager to get out and walk along the path by the river, I wrapped up warm and set off at about 11 a.m. I decided to try something April is encouraging us to do as a part of our writing course, which is to do a memory walk (walking when immersed in one's own thoughts and memories). This can be on your own or with a buddy. Today my buddy was my iPod which had the music of 'Les Mis' ringing in my ears. I plodded through the snow, stopping on occasions to watch the birds flying over the marshes searching for morsels of food and shelter. The snow blanketed the ground thickly and gave an eerie silence to the walk. The cathedral loomed high above the trees, giving an additional focus for my thinking.

25th January – Canterbury

A very pleasant journalist rang me today about an article she wants to write about me in a *Your Health* magazine article for East Kent. We also fixed a date for a photographer to visit me to take photographs to accompany the piece. We have agreed the article will be entitled 'I'm still me: Living with dementia' with the sub-heading 'Dementia doesn't define me'.

30th January – London

I co-presented with Gaynor Smith an Alzheimer's Society service user involvement training workshop at the Wesleyan chapel. Rosemary came up to London with me and took the opportunity to head off and explore the area round about, particularly the shops in the vicinity of Angel and Old Street.

I enjoy planning and delivering these training sessions. It's really part of my comfort zone, because it takes me back to being a teacher once again. Amongst the 16 delegates were Alzheimer's Society staff who are keen to become champions of service user involvement. They will use the training to cascade the message to colleagues.

After the event, Rosemary and I met up with Julian Washington, who is the son of Marlene, one of my deputies from Blean.

8th February – Herne Bay

Travelled with Elizabeth Field to help deliver a talk on living well with dementia to a group of people recently diagnosed. I found it interesting talking to the group both collectively and individually. I was also able to give them some insight into what dementia has been like for me, and to share with them some of the coping strategies that I've been able to develop.

13th February – London

My first visit with Reinhard to the British Psychological Society's headquarters in Tabernacle Street. This was a conference organised by the society, and my role was to talk about me the person, my diagnosis and life afterwards.

Because of the professional audience, I was keen to explore and talk with them about the benefits of a diagnosis, and how I feel post-diagnostic support can be improved.

Sharing the agenda with me was Dawn Brooker, who gave a very good talk about informed consent and pre-diagnostic counselling, using the analogy of a river. I've never really thought about pre-diagnostic counselling, seeking to focus on what happened after the diagnosis. It caused me to think back to my assessment, and the support that Elizabeth Field gave me during that assessment process which enabled me to better deal with what was happening at the time. Amongst other speakers were Daniel Collerton and Sue Watts, both of whom I met through Reinhard.

15th February – Canterbury

I've really enjoyed the writing course at the university, and this is the final session today. The group are extremely able writers and very enthusiastic.

I kept from the group the fact that I had dementia until the latter stages of the course, because I wanted to be treated as an equal and not to be treated any differently. This seemed to work.

The writing from the group is of such a high standard that, with April Doyle's leadership, we have all chosen to submit work for a group anthology to be published later. I have offered two pieces, like most of the group; one of mine is about a significant character from my childhood, Uncle Joe, and the other is a reflective piece about Christmases in my past.

16th February – Canterbury

I'm finding shopping more and more difficult, to the point where I now prove a challenge to Rosemary when we go shopping in the supermarket. It's far better now that she does this on her own, without the encumbrance of me wandering off, or picking up things from the shelves and putting them in the trolley when she's already got them. Whilst she shops now, I'm developing my vacuuming skills at home...

19th February–31st March – Adelaide, Australia

Before departing in a taxi late in the afternoon for Heathrow, Rosemary and I went to a morning meeting at the Conservative Club in Canterbury with Canterbury's MP Julian Brazier. This was through our EKIDS group and I was keen to share with him something about what living with dementia is like and to give him a sense of the group.

Six weeks this time in Australia! We are so lucky to have this opportunity, and to think if we had taken the neurologist's advice three years ago we would have missed out on five more trips to our beloved Oz. No yellow brick road leading there, but with 'Meet and Assist', a sympathetic supportive airline and airport is a good substitute!

Whilst we as always enjoyed the lovely company of long-established

Aussie friends it was also a great pleasure to meet up for a meal with Australian activist and writer Kate Swaffer and her husband Pete on their 'home patch'. We also visited the HQ of the Alzheimer's Association in Adelaide with our dear friend Hellen for an informative talk by Christian Bakker, from the Netherlands, about young onset dementia. Both Rosemary and I were most impressed by what Christian outlined as provision for younger people with dementia in his country.

I'm reminded of the fact when travelling back from Australia that in 2008 I was starting a new job – the advisory role in Maidstone – on the very day that we landed from Adelaide. Alf, who at the time did the return taxi journeys to Heathrow, had to do a detour on our return to drop me off in Maidstone to start the new job, and then take Rosemary home with the luggage. It caused quite a stir within the advisory team when we were asked to speak about where we'd travelled from to the meeting that day. One person was quite impressed that she'd travelled down from London to Maidstone for the meeting: that was slightly trumped by me saying I'd come from Adelaide!

12th–15th April – Eastbourne
We so look forward to these annual Shepherdswell WI trips and this one was slightly blighted by a very wet Saturday in Brighton, but made up for by a sunny Sunday strolling along the esplanade and pier in Eastbourne. I followed this with half an hour browsing around an enormous second-hand bookshop in the town.

18th April – Dartford
I have been nominated for the KMPT Volunteer of the Year award. Consequently today, Rosemary and I went to the awards ceremony in Dartford. Having no anticipation of winning, and indeed, feeling rather flattered and slightly embarrassed at being nominated, I decided we would meet with Rosemary's sister Barbara and her husband, Michael, to enjoy the day with them by having a meal in a pub. This lessened for me any sense of worry or pressure about the evening.

When it came to the ceremony, I was really surprised to win the award.

On the journey home I have been reflecting upon the award, and whilst very grateful for the recognition and humbled by the faith placed in me, I do feel a growing sense of pressure and expectation around my abilities. This makes me uneasy and reinforces a sense of 'unworthiness' around the accolades and plaudits that some people crave.

19th April – Canterbury

Our service user network group has now been running for five months, and has only just decided upon its name. We're to be called the Kent Forget Me Nots (because we're aware that there are other groups called 'Forget Me Nots' around the country). Today was our monthly meeting, and we were delighted to be joined by Nada Savitch, who came down from Innovations in Dementia in London. Reinhard, Nada and I went for a pre-meeting lunch in Canterbury. I have discovered that Innovations consists of three ex-Alzheimer's Society employees – Nada, Rachael Litherland and Steve Milton. They have formed a small organisation seeking to advance the involvement of people with dementia. If the other two are anything like Nada, I am looking forward to meeting and working alongside them.

Numbers within our Forget Me Nots group have gradually increased, and apart from two people dropping out because of their advancing dementia no one has left the group. If you offer they will come, if they contribute they will stay, is for me the axiom here.

29th April – Canterbury

Every Wednesday for some time now I have been going into Wincheap Primary School to hear readers, and today I had one of those magical moments with an eight-year-old reader whose name is Lewis.

Lewis is a bright lad, and was taking his turn to come out into the corridor to read to me. He did so today with a bright, beaming smile on his face. His opening line to me was, 'I saw you in a magazine in my doctor's!' This is because the *Your Health* magazine has now been published and is being distributed via GP surgeries, clinics and pharmacies in the area – the article is the one headed 'Dementia doesn't define me'.

I had not spoken to the children about me having dementia; as far as they were concerned I was the retired head from Blean who comes in each week to hear them read. Preparing myself to get involved in a conversation with an eight-year-old about dementia, I braced myself to receive his next comment. Still smiling, he said, 'And I know your first name!'

Clearly, as far as Lewis was concerned, dementia didn't define me. He was defining me not just by the label 'Mr Oliver', which is how they refer to me, but by my first name as well! If only all adults would use one's name as the most appropriate label.

11th May – London

A wonderful day spent today in the company of Rosemary at the Savoy Hotel, where we were so privileged to meet actor Carey Mulligan and screenwriter Julian Fellowes. This event was organised by the Alzheimer's Society to mark the start of Dementia Awareness Week and was filmed for *Channel 4 News*.

One of the society's staff coordinating the event and engaging with the celebrities and families present was Jane Cotton. She is lovely, and both Rosemary and I sensed an immediate connection and sense of friendship with Jane. As daughter of Bill Cotton, who is famous for his work at the BBC, including bringing to prominence Morecambe and Wise and the Two Ronnies, and granddaughter of the voice of my Sunday lunchtimes as a child – Billy Cotton – she is well placed in the company we shared today.

15th May – Canterbury

I had been invited to attend a staff meeting at Wincheap School to talk about dementia with the teachers, and to bring along with me some children's books, loaned to me for this purpose by the Alzheimer's Society, which are written about dementia for families to use. Reinhard was happy to come along to support me, so we did a double-act with the staff. This was interesting because, in a sense, our roles were being reversed: this was more familiar territory for me than for Reinhard, even though his youngest son goes to that school.

17th May – Canterbury

A very positive first annual review of the envoy role at St Martin's Hospital today. In attendance in addition to myself were Reinhard, Janet Lloyd and Jon Parsons, one of the directors of KMPT. Everyone agreed that we should carry on for at least another year.

28th May – Canterbury

Rosemary and I this evening went along to Thanington Resource Centre to support the group managing the Hambrook Marshes, who were holding their annual general meeting (AGM). There was an interesting talk alongside the AGM about the wildlife of the marshes, with particular focus on bees. I think the intention is to set up some hives within the marshes to encourage bees.

30th May – London

Reinhard and I have had an invite from the Dementia Engagement and Empowerment Project (DEEP) and the Mental Health Foundation to meet with Mike Howarth, an ex-dentist from Manchester, and some professionals who are supporting him. Mike is, I guess, about 80 years old, and is working for the Trust part time in the Salford area, doing similar work to myself in raising awareness about what living with dementia is like. The brief for this meeting was to explore through DEEP how employers can better help employees who are living with dementia to carry on working, and part of the outcome of this will be to produce a DEEP guide.

1st June – Canterbury

Having read Melvyn Bragg's new book, *Grace and Mary*, which is fiction loosely based on the story of his mother who had dementia, I went to Waterstones in Canterbury today to get the book signed by the author. I had an engaging conversation with Melvyn Bragg about dementia, during which he was interested to note that I had it, and how young I am, and that I don't look like a 'typical person with dementia'. He also showed interest in finding out more about the galantamine that I'm taking.

4th June – Canterbury

As part of our attendance at Canterbury's Ideal Spine Centre, Rosemary and I attended a juicing workshop, and subsequently have bought a juicer. We're now going to try a juice diet for a week to see the potential health benefits. Health professionals can help, as indeed can friends, but everyone also needs to take some responsibility for their own health for as long as is possible.

7th June – Maidstone

I presented a paper today to the KMPT Young Onset Dementia Network with Reinhard. The paper was about comparing services and support for young onset dementia in Australia, the UK and the Netherlands, based on mine and Rosemary's recent trip to Australia and a talk we heard given by a Dutch clinician named Christian Bakker at the offices of the Australian Alzheimer's Association.

11th June – London

Recently I've been invited to join a project advisory group as part of an occupational therapy project entitled VALID, which stands for Valuing Active Life in Dementia. This is an extremely interesting long-term project seeking to introduce a substantial programme of occupational therapy into dementia care within our NHS system, based on a model developed in the Netherlands. There is an interesting parallel there with the young onset dementia talk I gave a few days ago to the Young Onset Dementia Network.

Whilst I was at VALID, which meets in the Friends Meeting House near Euston, Rosemary came with me and used the opportunity of the meeting to have a walk and explore that vicinity.

12th June – Canterbury

Having been interviewed a week ago by a journalist from the *International Business Times* (IBT), today the article was published. It followed a contact from Dementia UK who had picked up an article in the national press about a man who had been diagnosed with dementia, and fairly soon afterwards had found this too difficult to live with and so had consequently committed suicide. The IBT wanted my view on this, and Dementia UK wanted me to portray a more positive approach.

The brief was that this man had felt the diagnosis was a fate worse than death. I was asked the question, do I see it as such? My answer was a straightforward 'no'. Suicide doesn't have to follow diagnosis. Although there are foggy days, they are a mixture of subtle and wretched. The journalist asked me what I did on foggy days, to which I said (and he quoted me back on this), 'I think, sod dementia, and I go out into the garden and spend some time out there to restore the sun in my life.'

Well, the journalist latched onto this and produced a really good article, but with a headline that concerned me: 'Sod dementia, says dementia sufferer'. I spoke to him about this a couple of days ago, before publication, and he agreed to take out the word 'sufferer', but wouldn't remove the expletive: he felt it was eye-catching. So from now on I will try to make light of it, and forever more it will be called the 'Sod dementia article'.

It taught me that working with the press, I'll win some and I'll lose some. But at least in this case we did arrive at a compromise.

15th June – Menton, France

Again, with the luxury of using Kent's Manston Airport, we flew to Genoa, and then transferred by coach across the border into France for a very pleasant and restful week's holiday on the Mediterranean coast. One highlight for us was being able to explore the riches of Provence, and to see that beautiful countryside bedecked in purple from lavender fields.

28th June – London

Reinhard and I have been invited to attend the young onset dementia conference at University College London (UCL), organised by the Mental Health Sciences Unit at UCL in association with Dementia Care. I was not speaking, but sat in the audience with Reinhard.

In fact, there were no service users speaking or involved in the agenda. It was solely a professional list of speakers, amongst whom was Raymond Koopmann from the Netherlands. Professor Koopmann is the head of the centre where Christian Bakker works and he elaborated upon the fascinating care work around young onset dementia they are doing in Nijmegen. It seems to me that the Netherlands has featured very strongly in the events that I've attended thus far in 2013.

Although there were some good speakers and interesting pieces, including one by Jacqui Hussey in which she outlined a model that was being developed in Wokingham, both Reinhard and I felt frustrated by the fact that there was a general sense within the conference of being done 'to' and 'for' people with dementia rather than being done 'with'.

2nd July – Maidstone

Daren Kerle took me to Maidstone Library to hear support for Kent County Council's application for a national award linked to the work that we've done together in helping people with dementia access services such as libraries, museums and art galleries in the county. We will await the decision of the judges. I was able to spend time speaking to the judges, explaining to them my role within the work.

Another positive today was that Mycal Miller, who made the film about me for the council, was there. It was good to catch up.

5th July – Canterbury

Having been to a number of post-diagnostic groups with Elizabeth Field in Herne Bay and Folkestone, today's was at St Martin's Hospital in Canterbury. I felt it would be good to take someone else along to build up more people's experience of delivering at these events, so today Tony from the Forget Me Nots group came along too.

Tony is not used to speaking in public to audiences and, with mine and Elizabeth's help, was able to give a different perspective about living well with dementia, which was appreciated by the audience.

I've been reflecting recently about the fact that, ever since I was a child, I've been treated as if I were older than my years. I guess being tall, and possibly being quite a bright child, contributed to this. Now, here I am, in my 50s, at times being treated – because of the dementia – as if I'm in my 70s. An irony there, I feel.

6th July – Romney, Hythe and Dymchurch Railway

Today was the third annual EKIDS trip. We joined the railway in Hythe and a group of about ten of us travelled by steam train through Dymchurch and Romney to the terminus at Dungeness. It was a very hot day, and whilst the conversation was good, we could have done with getting off and stretching our legs during the journey.

One claim to fame for Dungeness is that it's Britain's only desert, and on a day when the temperature exceeded 30 degrees, that's pretty much what it felt like! It is overlooked by the immense nuclear power station, and apart from the 'greasy spoon' café and the plants fighting the elements to survive on the beach, the best feature for me was exploring the fascinating garden of Derek Jarman, who passed away some years ago with AIDS.

10th July – Middlesex

At a recent Forget Me Nots meeting Sarah Ghani, a clinical psychologist from West London, came to speak to us. At the end of the meeting she invited Reinhard and me to go to her Trust to speak at a conference being organised today.

The brief for Reinhard and me was to speak about effective user involvement, in order that Sarah could help inspire people within her Trust to support this, and also to come forward as volunteers to lead it. Other speakers at the event included Professor Craig Ritchie, who led a piece of research in dementia, part of his focus being to examine the James Lind Alliance's ten key priority areas for research to be recommended and followed by the Alzheimer's Society.

15th July – Margate

Today Reinhard, Carolina (a Forget Me Nots member) and I, along with Jen, a psychologist from Thanet, interviewed four candidates for a post of assistant psychologist based partly in Thanet and partly in Dover. This was a much better experience than my former experience of interviewing with KMPT. We were all unanimous in our choice, and Ian Asquith got the job.

17th July – Gravesend to London

A sweltering hot day for our trip with the U3A on the *Pocahontas*, sailing from Gravesend along the Thames to the centre of London. This was a trip I really had wanted to do for some time, and both Rosemary and I thoroughly enjoyed it. There was actually an extra bonus that before we boarded the boat, because the coach arrived early in Gravesend, we were able to make a diversion to see the Sikh temple in Gravesend, which is really quite magnificent.

19th July – Canterbury

The Forget Me Nots group meets on the second Friday of every month. We always begin our meeting with a round-the-table item to ensure that each member has at least one opportunity to speak if they so wish. We always choose a theme and a topic for this item on the agenda, and it seems to be well received and well supported. Today was a particularly enjoyable one, when each person with dementia, supporter and professional there was invited to bring along a favourite piece of poetry to read. I chose 'Please Mrs Butler' by Allan Ahlberg, which was always a favourite of mine when teaching and as a head. Another Forget Me Not who chose a memorable piece for me was Melvyn, who picked a poem by Siegfried Sassoon, one of the World War I poets.

Feeling quite well at present, possibly aided by being on a juice diet for a week as recommended by Christian Farthing.

23rd July – Canterbury

Professor Jan Dewing, who replaced Penny at the dementia centre within Canterbury Christ Church University, visited me at home today to establish a link, and to discuss the possibility of me planning and delivering a public lecture at the university on living with dementia. This will launch a series of health talks at the university in the autumn.

Through the Alzheimer's Society today I was telephoned by the *Reader's Digest* for an interview with me which will be published this September. We agreed that the theme for the article would be my story around dealing with the diagnosis and then showing how I am trying to live as well as is possible with my dementia.

2nd August – Canterbury

A special workshop today at Thanington of the Forget Me Nots supported by the British Psychological Society and the Dementia Action Alliance to formulate two guidebooks on post-diagnostic support which could be used to support people with dementia and professionals.

This action of those three organisations working together reminds me of a quote from Tony Benn, who said, 'Protest doesn't work, only demand does.' He used as examples apartheid and the Suffragettes. We now do need to demand positive change in order to secure a level of post-diagnostic care and support which will be supportive of people living well. I'm gaining an increasing sense of a movement starting in trying to bring about change for people with dementia, and I very much want to be part of this change for the better in dementia care.

5th August – Canterbury

Gaynor Smith visited me at home with a freelance photographer to discuss issues linked to service user involvement within the Alzheimer's Society and to give the photographer an opportunity to take pictures of me in my home environment, which could be banked by the society for use in publications later.

16th August – Canterbury

Combined DEEP and Forget Me Nots meeting to work on a range of DEEP guides around involving people with dementia after their diagnosis. I get confused, but it seems to me that DEEP stands for Dementia Engagement and Empowerment Project, and whilst others are involved, key players from where I am sitting are Nada, Rachael and Steve from Innovations.

18th–22nd August – Nottingham

Went to see my mother in the care home to celebrate her 81st birthday with her. There was evidence of cheerful banter and positive relationships between her and the care home staff looking after her, which was good to see. We are still feeling quite frustrated though by the fact that, despite labelling her clothes with her name, when we visit her sometimes a number of those items can't be found. Also she still often asks me, 'When is Lew [my dad] coming to see me?' She sometimes does not remember that he died three years ago. I want to be honest with her but also do not want to open up the grieving process again, so my response is, as usual, 'He won't be coming today.' This pacifies her and, whilst honest, of course the full picture is that he won't ever be visiting her again. I think it was Maya Angelou who wrote, 'When people speak with brutal honesty, what is most remembered is the brutality, not the honesty.' I totally agree.

29th August – Canterbury

I was filmed at home again by Mycal Miller, accompanied today by Julia Burton-Jones. They are putting together a financial bid for Dementia Pathfinders to support people with young onset dementia after diagnosis.

Dementia Pathfinders was formed after the restructuring of Dementia UK, and because of the individuals involved, I'm happy to be part of that organisation and support it with my name and my time. With regard to the filming, it was interesting to note how much harder I found it a year on after previously filming with Mycal. We had to do many more takes and I got frustrated with myself, sensing I hadn't done such a good job.

Mycal was even more patient, sensitive and supportive, which enabled me to complete the piece.

30th August – Canterbury

I've been approached by Channel 4 to be one of five advisors on a new TV series looking at dementia care. I'm the only person who is not an eminent academic from the dementia world. Today I was visited by the series producer Gayl Paterson to discuss the concept for the programme and what my role might be in it.

I don't want to be filmed, because I don't think that my story is relevant to people at the stage that the programme is focusing on. Where I feel I can be of help is in an advisory role, and Gayl is more than happy with this.

2nd September – London

I attended the DAA quarterly meeting at the Royal Pharmaceutical Society with Reinhard. The main items on the agenda today were talks about delirium, cultural elements of dementia care, and the carers' call to action, the latter led by Rachel Niblock.

6th September – Canterbury

After experiencing some issues in finding a room at St Martin's Hospital this afternoon, I met the seven students on placement this year. This year's cohort is really well prepared, engaging and enthusiastic. They and I did the same exercise that Mycal had shown me at the library workshop around asking people to record something from their past, present and future. This unearthed some useful information about the group as individuals which will be helpful in getting to know each other. Another key message I want to convey to them, and health professionals generally, is how we can support each other through getting to know the person – something from their life story, their current situation and their future hopes and aspirations – including those with dementia!

I think the students I am most likely to work closest with are Alex and Lewis, who are based in Dover with Reinhard, and Sophie, Charley and Jen, who are in Canterbury.

9th September – Canterbury

Visited at home today by Australian lecturer Kim Robinson from Kent University, who is delightful. We spent time chatting both about Australia and her request that I help her on the social studies course at the Medway campus.

10th September – Canterbury

Spoke at an event today with Tanya Clover at St Martin's, supported by Laura who works at Kent County Council as part of the Dementia Friendly Communities team. I took along with me the mask I'd made at Christ Church University, and the DVD from the film with Mycal. I used them to form a talk around my hopes and fears, my story, and what I feel living in care *might* be like, *could* be like and *should* be like when that time arrives. Tanya and I also gave our individual perspective on the work of Tom Kitwood.

I am now devoting more time and thought to the importance of the 'Kitwood flower' and how useful it is, with regard not only to dementia care but also to living in what we would wish to be a caring society.

17th September – Canterbury

I have been invited by Professor Jan Dewing to launch the autumn season of public lectures, and today's went really well. I was given a 90-minute slot in the lecture theatre to quite a large audience, some of whom I knew. In the audience alongside Rosemary were the current year's students, Ian Asquith and Reinhard. Some colleagues from Blean and Dover came to support, and also a large number of health professionals, some of whom I recognised.

Today's talk coincided with the publication of the *Reader's Digest* magazine with the article about me in it.

Although preparing and writing talks is getting harder, often the hardest thing about the process is deciding which shirt to wear! I really go into the zone and feel comfortable with doing the talks. I am, to an extent, oblivious to the surroundings and people in the room with me. The title of today's talk was 'This is me – dementia and my life'.

I do often find the questions and answers section hard, and there was one that caught me out today. I can't remember what the question was, but I do remember feeling thrown by it.

18th September – Canterbury

This morning, Rosemary told me that in the night I'd been speaking in a foreign language in my sleep. She couldn't work out what it was, but she thought it wasn't French. This somewhat alarmed us both as I have not, as far as I know, done anything like this before.

20th September – Canterbury

A number of the Forget Me Nots joined a DEEP advisory meeting hosted locally. We were being supported by our students on placement, and amongst the members of the advisory group were representatives from the Mental Health Foundation, Comic Relief, a number of universities, Innovations in Dementia, the Alzheimer's Society, and a gentleman named Peter Ashley who I've seen previously at Dementia Action Alliance meetings in London, and who I know is a longstanding and particularly well-respected person with dementia advocating for the cause.

I am currently reading *Me Talk Pretty One Day* by American writer David Sedaris, which was recommended to me by my writing tutor, April Doyle. Amongst what I am taking from the book is a desire not to hurt or alienate anyone I know through what I write. Also, I hope, to raise a few smiles.

26th September – Reading

Gaynor and I delivered the service user training for the first time outside of London. This was to reach a wider audience than just those who are London based or able to travel into the city. To support me on this occasion, Rosemary and our daughter Karon came along, and whilst I was delivering the workshop, they went off and explored some of the delights and shops that Reading has to offer.

The training went well; it was a different venue, a different group of people, but giving the same messages around the importance of service user involvement, and it taught practical ways to achieve this effectively.

27th September – Canterbury

A rarity for me, repeating a talk from last year, although, being me, I have to update and refine it – partly to freshen it up for myself, but also to make sure that the contents are relevant for the audience, and an accurate depiction of how and where I am currently with regard to coping with my dementia.

The audience today was third-year undergraduate occupational therapy students.

From time to time I ask the audience, if it's locally delivered, whether any of them know me from my previous existence as a teacher. I'm glad I did so today, because somebody put their hand up and said, 'Yes, Mr Oliver, you did teach me back in Swalecliffe in the 1990s,' so I was really pleased to meet up again with Ben, a former pupil.

30th September – Canterbury

I've started to record in my diary and calendar when I say no to dementia-related activities and invitations. Recently I've said no to the launch of the *Dementia Diaries* book in Maidstone, and no to an Innovations in Dementia media workshop in London. This is because I am getting asked to do more and more, and I need to be aware and conscious of the pressures that places not just on me, but also on Rosemary and/or my support network.

When being offered a particular project to be involved in, I have started to apply five criteria. First, can I make the date – is it free in my diary? Second, what will be the impact of saying yes on me and on Rosemary? Third, if I am attending with Rosemary, can we get there easily between us, and what will she feel about being part of the event that's taking place? If I'm going with a student supporter or with Reinhard, I'm conscious of leaving Rosemary behind, back at home. Fourth, what support will be available to enable me to get to the event and to then engage in the activity? Finally, what will be the impact on the piece of work? Is having me there a tokenistic gesture, or can I genuinely contribute to helping move the work forward?

8th October – Canterbury

Another welcome visit from Julia Burton-Jones from Dementia Pathfinders, who wanted to discuss with me a project called YODEL (Young Onset Dementia Engaged Living), which is connected to young onset dementia, and a book that Dementia Pathfinders are producing to support awareness-raising around young onset dementia.

Whilst waiting for Julia to arrive, Rosemary and I were doing our daily crossword puzzle from the *i* newspaper. We both derive a lot from this. On the foggier days, finding the answers is clearly more difficult, and even on the sunnier days there are times when my spelling frustrates me, and I am inclined now to repeat consonants and miss out vowels in words, which I find strange.

9th October – London

Reinhard, Lewis and I attended a conference at the British Psychological Society (BPS) to launch the documents that the Forget Me Nots and the BPS had worked on a couple of months ago. My involvement in the day was to speak about service user involvement, and the benefits that it can bring to the professionals and the person affected by dementia. Alongside that we explored the content of psychosocial interventions and their benefits, relating this to the work I do.

For some time I've been thinking about the emotional/cognitive balance, and how that is shifting for me, from being someone who was cognitively focused to now being much more influenced by my emotions. I find this to be both positive and negative. A year or two ago I read that Aristotle thought the heart was the location of one's intelligence; well, I hope that as my brain shrinks my heart grows!

At the end of the talk, Reinhard shared with me the evaluations of those who attended, and I am thrilled to see my talk scored 4.86 out of 5, which is so encouraging.

13th–22nd October – Canterbury

Keeping these nine days totally dementia-free, which included turning down seeing the Prime Minister at the G8 summit in London, alongside saying no to *BBC Breakfast* on the same subject. I need to focus upon decorating our bedroom and doing activities with the family.

At this time of year we seem to be inundated with spiders coming in from the garden to seek sanctuary from the cold. As a diversion from the decorating this inspired me to sit down and try in five minutes to produce a piece of creative writing, something which April was keen to encourage me to do but which I had stepped away from doing.

'The trap was set. The spider lurked, concealed by the petals of the rose and cunningly camouflaged by its chameleon-like qualities. Patience and hunger were his main drivers. Staring silently from his silken lair. Watching, waiting, thinking and motionless. How long had it been since his last meal had presented itself? He had no memory, no sense of time. In fact time stood as still as the spider himself. Would it be breakfast, lunch or dinner? It mattered not, all his thoughts were solely upon food. He had set the trap and into his world a fly had stumbled. Now was his chance. An opportunity not to be missed. A gourmet opportunity, tasty enough to stave off the hunger pangs he was feeling. Stealthily, for he knew he had to be careful, he silently and cautiously moved forward. The trap might work...'

30th October – Canterbury

Having spent a few days in my office getting back into the swing of the envoy role, Rosemary and I took a lovely diversion this evening by going to Shirley Hall in Canterbury to watch Adam Hills, the Australian comedian, who is a favourite of ours, perform stand-up as part of the Canterbury Festival.

14th November – Canterbury

Nada Savitch visited me at home for the first time. She came to write an article about the DEEP guides. To support this we had Alex Bone with us, one of this year's able placement students.

After they'd both left, I sat down and pondered upon what we'd produced during the day, and was left with many thoughts. Some say they 'fight' dementia – I try to outmanoeuvre and outwit it. I have never been aggressive or wished to fight anyone. At one time I subscribed to the sense of fighting for a cause – I now feel that I think and talk for the causes I hold dear. The pen is mightier than the sword.

18th November – Canterbury

Noted today that the film Mycal Miller and I made in August 2012 has now been on YouTube for eight months, and has passed 800 views.

When Mycal put the film on YouTube, I remember emailing him being quite celebratory of the fact that we'd passed 50 views, and then astonished when the figure reached a hundred. Now, here we are, approaching a thousand! I wonder how many more times the film will be watched and, indeed, who is watching it, and of what benefit it is to them.

20th November – London

Following our writing session last week Alex and Nada supported me in speaking at the DAA annual event at Westminster Hall. I think the grandiose surroundings of the venue lifted me to perform at my very best. I was helping launch the DEEP guides. The guides were informed by a Forget Me Nots meeting I co-led recently, and cover areas such as setting up and running groups for and with people with dementia, tips for employers who want to be more dementia-friendly, and language to use when referring to people with dementia. I am sure the intention is to produce more in the future. The feedback from the event included words like 'inspirational'.

I've had many plaudits and praises in the past couple of years since taking on the role of envoy and speaking about dementia. This is one of the first occasions I can remember that the word 'inspirational' has been attached to me. Whilst that is humbling and positive to hear, it comes with a tinge of embarrassment and uncertainty as to whether it's a fitting label to attach to me.

During the talk I was reminded of a story I read in a book written by Martin Sheen and his son Emilio Estevez called *Along the Way*. In the book, an old Irish story is told. There's an old man about to enter into heaven, and St Peter stops him at the Pearly Gates. St Peter asks the man to show his scars before being allowed to enter into heaven. The man hesitates and says, 'But I have no scars,' to which St Peter replies, 'Was there nothing worth fighting for?'

I relate this story to the mask of mine, which I remember noting in my diary. Doing the voluntary work that I do does indeed give me a great sense of satisfaction, but does at times come with a cost, and that cost brings scars.

But it IS worth fighting for.

26th November – London

Being part of the Alzheimer's Society Research Network, today I attended a panel meeting supported by Sophie, one of this year's students. The panel is newly established and reflects the splitting of the Alzheimer's Society research portfolio into bio-chemical, care, services and public health. I have allied myself to the latter because that's where I feel I can be most useful and most effective.

28th November – Medway

Following the visit to my home recently by lecturer Kim Robinson from the university, today Alex drove me to Chatham to attend a teaching session with social sciences undergraduates as part of their course about user involvement. My talk was entitled 'This is me', my aim being to increase the students' understanding of dementia.

4th December – London

Had the privilege this evening of speaking at the Alzheimer's Society inaugural Christmas carol service at St Paul's Church in Knightsbridge, supported by Rosemary alongside Caroline Davy and Jane Cotton from the Alzheimer's Society. Amongst others there speaking and in the audience were Carey Mulligan, Tony Robinson, Angela Rippon, Kevin Whately and Sharon Maughan, who is the actress wife of Trevor Eve.

I talked with Tony Robinson about archaeology programmes on TV including but also beyond *Time Team*, and about *Lewis* with Kevin Whately, all of which was very interesting. The highlight though for me was a great conversation with Carey about films and music from the 1960s, which is the background to her new film, *Inside Llewyn Davis*. I am so looking forward to seeing this in the new year when it is released. The warmth of our conversation was captured by the society's photographer who was taking shots as we talked and laughed heartily.

The subject for my talk was based upon anecdotes from Christmas in school, and one of the audience asked me if it was inspired by Gervase Phinn, to which I said, 'No – it was inspired by my own experience' – but I could understand the parallels with those written about by Gervase Phinn.

At the end of my talk I read as a poem the words of the song 'While I Am Here' by Eric Bogle, which I guess is becoming a signature tune for me as I use it so often at talks I deliver. The lyrics of the song mean so much to me.

5th December – Canterbury

Following an approach from ITV South East news, today I was filmed at my home. Their original concept for the piece was to film me doing something that I used to be able to do, and now cannot do it as well. I said I wouldn't even consider it. If they wanted to come to my home to film me, they'd have to film me doing something competently now, or showing a new skill that I'm trying to develop. They agreed to this, and the piece, I thought, was good.

To give me additional support, I called upon Reinhard, who needed to look after his son at the time that the film crew had arranged. He asked if he could bring him along as well, which I gladly agreed to. They interviewed

Reinhard, and then they filmed his son playing with Lego®, so he got to be on television too!

7th–9th December – Nottingham

Visited my mum with Rosemary in her care home. She seems not so good at the moment, and her dementia is affecting her more and more with each visit. She understandably hates being hoisted due to her lack of mobility which means that she fears needing the toilet. So she drinks very little, and then develops urinary infections and becomes dehydrated.

13th December – Medway and Canterbury

Having spoken to undergraduates last month at the Medway site with Alex, today both of us returned to the same campus, this time to speak to master's post-graduate students who are on the social studies course. Consequently, I revised the talk considerably and made it more appropriate for students at this stage of their studies, providing them with much more depth and much greater breadth of understanding. The focus again was living with dementia and the challenges that dementia presents, alongside coping strategies and how to involve people with dementia in social services.

It was interesting today to meet Jocelyne Kenny, a trainee clinical psychologist studying at Royal Holloway, part of London University. This is the same university our daughter Karon attended and then got married at.

Jocelyne came to speak to the Forget Me Nots about her doctoral thesis, which is around people being involved in services and living with dementia. I understand Jocelyne had attended a previous meeting of the group, but I'm afraid I had little recall of that, so it was good to spend a little bit longer today getting to know her and the work that she's seeking to do.

17th December – Brentford

Having spoken to the *Sunday Times* recently about a major research project called PREVENT, which is seeking to identify potential risks to people in their 40s and 50s of developing dementia, today I attended a monitoring meeting on behalf of the Alzheimer's Society. This is designed to monitor the project and then to report back to Matt at the Alzheimer's Society

Research Network. There is a major amount of funding going into the project, and it will run from December 2013 to the autumn of 2016 with a two-year follow-up.

The project is constructed around two large groups of people. One group is people at higher risk of developing dementia because there may be a familial link, and the other is people who are low risk. It will examine their fitness and diet, test them and scan them, and then analyse the data to see whether there's any conclusions that can be drawn. From this, recommendations will be drawn around actions that can be put in place to – as the name of the project suggests – prevent the onset of dementia.

20th December – Canterbury

Had my first meeting today with Liz Jennings, whose name was given to me by Elizabeth Field as someone who is interested in helping with a writing project that is swirling around in the back of my mind involving people with dementia. This was inspired by the writing course I did with April Doyle, and I would like to consider how we can possibly capture some of that and use it to support people with dementia in learning to do life writing.

21st–30th December – Canterbury

My birthday and Christmas! As a child, having a birthday close to Christmas was not great. Often I would receive a combined present, and the two key days in a child's life for me were gone in a blink of an eye! Now each birthday I do look forward to the family gathering with us and often I receive book tokens from our adult children. I so enjoy browsing in bookshops – they are the only shops I go in with any sense of confidence these days, as even choosing and buying clothes on my own is beyond me. Then once books are bought I always read them; I read lots and remember very little, but whilst I was originally very frustrated by this I am now able to feel less so and take from a book the way it made me feel – a bit like a conversation with a person. I read every night before sleep for about 45 minutes, although if the book is about dementia I'll only read it during the day as it has in the past disturbed my sleep. I used to read history books and fiction; now my much reduced ability to remember facts and to follow plot and character steer me to reading only memoirs, which I do still enjoy.

31st December – Canterbury

A time for reflection. Whilst no outward celebration to mark New Year's Eve for me, the significance is that it is now three years since my diagnosis was confirmed. My life now is a bit like climbing mountains and looking at the view from the summit, alongside scrambling along pot holes into deep caverns which are dark and need a light shining to guide me along the slippery route. Having someone alongside me to navigate, encourage and support is crucial. I do feel life is being quite good to me whenever I am included in what is happening to me, for me and with me.

Sometime in 2013

Dear Alzheimer's

How can I see you as the enemy when you are part of me? I cannot fight you, in the long term I cannot beat you, but I will not cower or stay silent in your presence. Nor will I refrain from my best efforts to outwit you, and hopefully in my own small way I will try to inspire others to do likewise. I do still feel bulletproof, encased and protected by a shield of armour from your insidious advances, and allied to this I feel part of a movement of people, which enables me to feel involved, engaged, empowered and included. This may surprise you but you are actually becoming a force for positivity as you drive me into building up a presence and a constructive role.

One area where you and I wrestle is around the use of language. You will never define me and I will never be defined by you. I hate the word 'sufferer' and will never accept it. You see me as being the disease rather than having the disease. I am not demented, I have dementia – you don't have me! I am still the me in deMEntia.

I am fortunate that I can still leave you behind when going off on holiday, and during this year there have been some good examples of this, with travelling once again to Australia and breaking new ground by going to the South of France. I guess this surprises you?

The Forget Me Nots continue to grow in number, voice and influence, collectively and individually, and I know you fear this as a force to be reckoned with. Allied to this the students I work with as the next generation of professionals are being inspired by us to take lessons from the group and myself, and to use this as a platform to better serve those with dementia in order that others can live as well as possible whilst sharing their life with you.

The film I made in August will hopefully become a piece of work to illustrate how it is possible to live well with dementia. I know you hate to see those of us with dementia smiling. There is a lot of smiling in this film, although allied to the realism that life with you is not an easy ride, but there is hope and ways in which we can keep you at bay.

I am going to close now and take a rest, but before doing so I am going to remind you of a story I read recently and use in some of my talks. It is from *Along the Way* by Emilio Estevez and his father Martin Sheen, an actor and a human being who I admire greatly. The book tells the story of a man who has recently died and is about to try and enter through the gates of heaven. At the gates he is met by St Peter who stops the man and asks to see his scars before allowing him through. The man looks puzzled and replies, 'But I have no scars.' St Peter is sorry to hear this and responds with, 'Was there nothing worth fighting for?'

You have scarred me, dementia, but I am fighting you as this fight is certainly worth doing.

Yours insincerely

Keith

2014

—

'Welcome to my world'

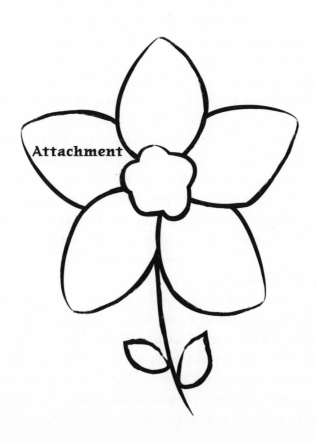

Attachment

5th January – Canterbury

I am sitting in my office today, after the Christmas break, ready to get back into the swing of things. Going through various emails, my eyes have been diverted to looking at the YouTube film that was placed by Mycal Miller on 27th April 2013, entitled *Keith Oliver's Story*. I'm now amazed to see that it has passed a thousand views, and I remember thinking how pleased and surprised I was when we passed 50, then a hundred. I never expected to reach anything like this sort of figure.

10th January – Canterbury

Today Liz Jennings came to visit the Forget Me Nots meeting to talk about the idea that she and I had discussed before Christmas of running a life writing course for people with dementia. In essence this was a follow-up to the Canterbury Christ Church University life writing course that I did last year with April Doyle. After we introduced and explained the idea to the group, we sent around a paper to ask who was interested, and approximately 12 people signed up, eight of whom seemed more committed and four described themselves as 'possibles'. We suggested that they went away after the meeting and thought more about this and chatted to their other halves. I know that a few people, such as Charles, had tried to get on the university course but had been unsuccessful, and here was an opportunity to do something fit for purpose for those with dementia. I am currently seeking support from the Alzheimer's Society, through Janet Baylis and other people at their headquarters, to achieve funding, which will allow us to employ Liz, to hire a venue and to support people with transport getting to and from each session. This is all new ground to me, and I feel excited but also very challenged by thinking about co-leading something like this.

14th January – London

Rosemary came to London with me today and saw me through to the venue for the Alzheimer's Society service user involvement training day being held at St Luke's, near Old Street. I was pleased that she was relaxed enough to go off and do some shopping in the vicinity nearby, and she rejoined us at the end of the session to sit in on the final elements of the day, before supporting me on the journey home. The session itself is around developing a workshop, which I'm increasingly confident about. The workshop will train Alzheimer's Society staff, starting with people who have identified themselves as potential champions for service user involvement within the society. As I felt well today, I was able to slightly deviate away from my script and add extra bits in, which seemed to make the day go better for myself and for participants.

15th January – London

I would never have thought a year or two ago that I would be invited to speak at a British Psychological Society conference. Today is a repeat of the event Reinhard and I attended in October with the students supporting us. This time, because the first event was oversubscribed, a repeat was being run, and Sophie came with Reinhard and me. What was different from last time is that today the new *Dementia Guide*, published by the Alzheimer's Society, the British Psychological Society and the DAA, was available for people to collect, and I was rather surprised to see a photograph of myself with the guide, sitting in our garden, as a means of advertising and promoting the guide. The conference went well again, and the feedback from participants was very good. As I felt less sure of myself today, I stuck pretty much to the original script.

21st January – Canterbury

Forget Me Nots Melvyn, Elizabeth and I, with Lewis Slade's support, attended a training day at our local hospital, the Kent and Canterbury. The event was for nursing staff, backup staff and hopefully some managers within the hospital, and the focus was very much upon dementia care in the acute hospital. Melvyn and I delivered a formal talk together, which was good, and then afterwards, informally, nurses came up to speak to us both. Many of them told us about how awful, at times, life in the hospital is for dementia patients, and also for staff trying their best to care for them. There was some uncertainty around one of my questions on staff training in dementia. It appears that between 8 and 20 per cent of ward staff in the three regional acute hospitals have had dementia training, and today will form a part of this. In addition, to deal with severe staff shortages, 31 additional nurses are being recruited from Spain, and all of them come with a level of dementia training. Elizabeth concluded the morning by speaking from the stage about the memory service.

23rd January – Herne Bay

Through Janet Britt, a friend and the secretary of the EKIDS charity, Rosemary and I went today to hear about the butterfly scheme, which is run in some hospitals throughout the country to support patients who are in general hospitals and who have dementia. The hospital Trust for this region does not invest in the butterfly scheme. It uses the *This Is Me* document published by the Alzheimer's Society. Both have many merits, but it appears from today's presentation that the butterfly scheme is much better. I asked myself the question, and then asked the question at the workshop, why is it not being used in our area, as it seems such a very good model? The only reason that one can arrive at is that there is a cost attached. We've seen a climate where, increasingly, we read in the newspapers about people with dementia spending time in hospital unnecessarily, and I'm sure this is an issue that isn't going to go away, and is probably going to get even more significant in time.

26th January–3rd March – South Australia

It's great that this time of year is being regarded as 'our time in Australia'. Usually the temperature for our stay remains in the mid-30s but this year it topped this with four days over 40 degrees, peaking at a record-breaking 45 on 2nd February. This is too hot even for stalwarts like us. All we could do on that day was head for the air-conditioned cinema and cool down with winter scenes in the film *The Book Thief*. I loved the book a couple of years ago and the film was very good also. Since 2010 we have avoided internal flights and independent travel within South Australia or inter-state. However, this year, because we have both been keeping quite well, we decided to be more adventurous, more like our old selves, and flew to Port Lincoln on the Eyre Peninsula and explored a region which we had never visited previously. Port Lincoln, by South Australian standards, is a reasonable-sized town. The narrow streets restrict the speed of cars to 20 km/h which gives the place a sleepy, slow and small feeling compared to British towns, and the airport was tiny – no baggage reclaim, just a trolley from off the plane, and the pre-flight aircraft check was conducted by the pilot and centred upon him kicking the tyres in front of the 30 passengers about to board to check they were up to take-off and landing.

12th March – Ashford

Having taken a week or so after our trip to Australia to get over jet lag, today was the first event in my diary connected to dementia. The event was to attend the KMPT Young Onset Dementia conference in Ashford, organised by Reinhard, and supported by Alex, one of the placement students. The aim of my talk today was to illustrate how it is possible, with support, to live well with young onset dementia, and to try to expand the knowledge of the audience around this issue. I chose to start my talk by showing some film footage of Torvill and Dean doing their amazing gold medal-winning ice dance to the *Boléro*. Whilst I went to primary school with Jane, this was not the reason I used this. In fact, Ravel composed that piece of music when experiencing young onset dementia himself. I then made the point of how often the medical world and the world in general write people off once diagnosed with dementia; here was another illustration of the opposite viewpoint. Staying creative, I then used Eric Bogle's lyrics to 'While I Am Here', talking through the significance of each verse, and built the rest of the talk around this, using my knowledge and experience from the Forget Me Nots to show that it's not just me – there are other people with young onset dementia who can take on an activist role alongside me.

20th March – Canterbury

This evening, a group of Forget Me Nots, professionals and students attended the Marlowe Studio in Canterbury to watch a play called *Finding Joy*. This was a dementia-focused play where actors wore masks to portray a story. I thought the performance was hard to follow, and I found the use of masks really quite disturbing. After the play, the students, Reinhard, Elizabeth, myself, Charles and Pauline remained in the auditorium with a number of other people whilst the actors came out on stage and did a Q&A with us. They were quite surprised to hear that there were people with dementia within the audience. I reflected upon this in conversation with Reinhard, Elizabeth and Alex in the pub nearby afterwards and came to the conclusion that the actors' surprise was brought about because they wondered either why we would wish to watch a play about the subject or how we could possibly be in a theatre after 9.30 in the evening. Maybe we educated and challenged them as much as they did us.

25th March – London

I co-delivered the Alzheimer's Society service user involvement training day again. It was very similar to the one that Gaynor Smith and I did a couple of months ago. This time, it was at Devon House. Alex, one of the students, came with me today, and she participated for the day as a member of the Alzheimer's Society staff by joining in the workshop, which worked well for her and certainly gave something to the group that she was working in. Having initially made this training for people who were identified as champions of service user involvement, now Gaynor and I are looking to run it out for more staff in the society. Through this, it is felt that people with dementia will be far better engaged in the Alzheimer's Society, which will benefit the individual and the charity.

1st April – London

Back to Devon House again today, this time to attend a Research Network meeting – again, coincidentally, with Alex. As we arrived a little early at St Katharine Docks, she and I walked along Royal Mint Street nearby in order to try and find locations which had been given to us by Bev, our Australian friend, who was tracing her husband John's family history. Apparently, John's family migrated from that area in the 1840s. With Alex's help, I was able to find and photograph a few locations, and will now, over the next couple of days, email those to Bev, which I hope she'll find useful. After the end of the meeting, Alex supported me in a conversation with Janet Baylis, where we talked about finance from an Alzheimer's Society grant for the writing course that we're hoping to run very soon.

8th April – Canterbury

Following an initial meeting with Nada and Alex at my house on 11th March, today we did a concluding workshop at my house where we wrote an article for the *Journal of Dementia Care*. Areas we are covering revolve around my personal view of engagement and empowerment based upon a wide range of activities I have undertaken in the last year or so. Nada and Alex were very patient and attentive in drawing out of my thoughts around the Forget Me Nots group, my efforts in the envoy role and some suggestions from me to others both as service users and service providers around how involving people with dementia can be engaging and empowering for all.

10th April – Canterbury

Having secured the funding from DEEP, the teacher (Liz) and the venue (Beaney Library in Canterbury), today we started the life writing course. We have eight writers, all of whom have dementia, and five psychology students who are on placement with the Mental Health Trust – Alex, Lewis, Sophie, Charley and Jen. The proposal is to run this course every two weeks for six sessions. Beyond that I am open minded. It will be interesting to see what happens. Almost none of the writers have ever written like this before. Liz has not taught before, and the students have not supported a project in this depth before. We are all learning together, which is a positive feature of the project.

The first session was really enjoyable. Everyone came away buzzing and excited by what we are trying to do, but also quite challenged and certainly stimulated. Liz did a grand job, because one senses, and indeed one knows, that working with people with dementia and teaching is not her comfort zone.

16th April – Canterbury

Today I had a visit from Pamela Gordon from Channel 4, who has taken over as producer of the documentary series that they have asked me to help with as an advisor. Pamela, like her predecessor, is committed and enthusiastic towards the project, and came over really well in conversation with Rosemary and myself. Whilst there has been a change of personnel, the concept, structure and strategy for the series remains largely the same. Pamela was very receptive to my suggestions, and wants the series to be accurate and balanced in its portrayal of dementia. We reiterated my role as being the person with dementia on their team of advisors, and she noted down and seemed to take on board the suggestions I made, largely around the way dementia should be portrayed from the individual's point of view, be they professional or service user. When she left to return to London I reflected upon a sense of responsibility I seem to have acquired in this advisory virtual team – four leading professors from the world of dementia and me.

17th April – London

I attended an Alzheimer's Society research monitoring training, this time at Devon House, and supported by Rosemary. I was pleased that she felt confident enough to take herself off along the banks of the Thames and explore that area, joining me for a coffee at the end with our friend Jane Cotton in a nearby café.

22nd April – Canterbury

Although my mother has been unwell recently, it was a shock to receive a phone call in the middle of last night from her care home in Nottingham to tell me that she had died. This was totally unexpected, and will now set in motion a series of things which I need to do. For six months, her health has been much more up and down, and raised my anxiety level about her. Now I need to devote some attention to sorting out a plethora of arrangements and business. I have kept detailed notes from when my father died four years ago and I will try to apply the same systematic approach that saw me through the labyrinth of arrangements back then.

23rd April – London

Having had a sleepless night wondering whether I should attend, and then talking it through with Rosemary, we decided it was important to take up an invitation that was placed a few weeks ago for us to attend St James' Palace for the Alzheimer's Society awards. Michael Parkinson was MC, and it was wonderful to witness the award winners who have been involved in some amazing projects, both as individuals and teams, and to honour this prestigious event. I felt very privileged and relaxed to be a guest rather than a participant.

24th April – Canterbury

I have been looking forward to and preparing over the past week for the launch of the Kent Dementia Action Alliance at Canterbury Christ Church University. This was a dementia marketplace event, and I had been lined up to be the keynote, alongside which I shared a stint on the Forget Me Nots stand. I also accessed a Dementia Friends awareness session as a participant, with placement student Sophie. I was able to stay for the full day because it was from mid- to late morning until early afternoon, which gave me time beforehand and afterwards to do some phone calls regarding my mother. Talking of which, to add to my stress the hospital has advised me that they have lost her body somewhere on their site. I do need to go up to Nottingham soon. This is all getting too much, and I've planned to do so the day after tomorrow. The dementia activities are actually giving me a positive outlet and almost serve as a distraction from the emotions and the distress of dealing with my mother's death. If it was a sitcom it would almost be laughable, but it isn't, it is real life. I am also having a lot of difficulty securing the registration of her death. I was hoping to achieve this from Canterbury rather than making a special trip up to Nottingham to do so. When my father died Rosemary and I were able to use his council house to stay in during the period between his death and the funeral. Of course, as my mum was in a care home this is not possible. Still, I will overcome these challenges with the support of Rosemary, alongside maintaining my 'head teacher' mindset as best as I can to pick my way through this difficult time.

25th April – Canterbury

I was working on formulating timely diagnosis papers today with a group of Forget Me Nots as part of the British Psychological Society, plus Rachael Litherland. I was really touched to see a sympathy card from the Forget Me Nots and students, and was told by Reinhard that this had been orchestrated by the students, who clearly do care, and have a compassionate sense of what I'm going through at the moment because of the loss of my mother. I'm trying to present a professional public face by trying to focus on what needs to be done regarding my mother alongside diverting myself through some of the events and tasks connected to my envoy role, which I am finding helpful in dealing with the grief. Privately it is hard. I've made an appointment for tomorrow to go into Canterbury to speak to the registrar.

26th April – Canterbury

Supported by Rosemary, I had the meeting today with the registrar at the Beaney. Terribly complicated. Terribly stressful. It appears that, because Mother died in Nottingham, and I'm trying to register the death in Canterbury, despite what people had told me on the phone, this is even more problematic. So tomorrow, Rosemary and I will go up to Nottingham to try and sort this out. At least now the hospital tells me the body has been found. It's now almost a week since she died.

6th May – London

Everything seems to have gone quiet at the moment with regard to my mother. I'm in liaison with the vicar and with the funeral directors, and it appears that because of issues in Nottingham beyond my control there's no chance of the funeral taking place until 19th May. I have booked this date, which, in fact, is actually four weeks after her death. With nothing more I can do to speed arrangements along today, I attended a quarterly meeting of the DAA at the Royal College of Nursing with Lewis. The theme for the event was dementia care, and I spoke in support of Rachel Thompson from the Royal College on the 'Big Cs' – care, community, commitment, coordination and collaboration. In the afternoon I sat back and was able to listen and learn from experts talking about adaptations to buildings and physical environments to make them more dementia friendly.

14th May – Maidstone

This was an unusual event today, in the sense that it was a European-organised event around dementia self-sustaining communities, and there were speakers from the International Health Alliance. Myself and two relatively recent Forget Me Nots members, Carolina and Chris Norris, supported by Alex, went along to Maidstone and met up with Steve Milton from Innovations in Dementia to do a presentation about what living with dementia is like. We spoke on a programme alongside a heavily skewed professional line-up from the Netherlands, Germany, Scotland and Liverpool; indeed, surprisingly, we were the only local speakers there for this conference in Kent. We certainly livened it up with our presentation! It was a very good team approach between the five of us, and we were told afterwards that it was one of the highlights of the conference.

16th May – Ashford

Following mine and Melvyn's talk at Kent and Canterbury Hospital a few months ago, today I was invited to go to the Ashford International Hotel to speak to acute hospital staff working across all the East Kent University Hospital Trust, and I was supported today by Sophie. The conference was called '6 Cs'– care, compassion, courage, commitment, communication and competence – and I was asked to speak about compassion. I gave myself the task of preparing a piece entitled 'Compassion in healthcare'. I began my research for my talk by looking at what the word 'compassion' means, and the first words in the dictionary involved the use of sympathy. Now this puzzled me, and challenged me, because I don't want sympathy. What I want is empathy. I don't want people to feel sorry for me, I want people to help care for me, and to understand better what it is that I'm living with. There were about two hundred in the audience and I was the only non-professional speaking and the only slot which related to dementia during the day.

The three themes I spoke about were what it is like to live with dementia, how hospital care should be for patients with dementia, and the amazing Forget Me Nots. Sophie helped me write the talk last week and we included a section on 'SPACE': **STAFF** who are well trained and skilled in caring for people with dementia; **PARTNERSHIP** – hospital staff working alongside carers to meet the needs of the patient; **ASSESSMENT** – and early identification soon after admission of the needs of the person with dementia; **CARE PLANS** that are person centred and individualised; and **ENVIRONMENTS** that are dementia friendly. I challenged those present to consider how much of this they regularly address in their day-to-day working.

I had Sophie's support throughout the day, including joining me on stage to manage the PowerPoint, which along with the talk she had helped me to write. I was very pleased with the way the day went, helped by us both enjoying a very pleasant lunch in this four-star hotel.

18th May – Nottingham

Rosemary and I travelled to Nottingham today to meet the undertakers and the vicar in readiness for tomorrow's funeral. I can't write any more in my diary. Maybe the words will come later.

19th May – Nottingham

Mother's funeral took place today. Having sorted out all the business side of her affairs with the care home and with anyone else who needed to know, I feel I have dealt with the business side rather better than the emotional, and in the interim period between her dying and today, I have tried, with cousin Jane's help, to sort out the bits and pieces from her flat within the nursing home. Amongst these were a number of pictures, and I found it emotionally challenging to see my mother in my mind, and in these pictures, as the younger 'Mam' when she was in her 30s, and not the older person in her 80s, or even 70s, living with Alzheimer's. In those early photos she was always smiling and smartly dressed. Her intelligence and warmth shines through. The bipolar in her 40s robbed my mother of much of her youthful exuberance which I benefited from as a child, and Alzheimer's robbed her of her memory and her mobility, but neither took away her spirit. There was always a vulnerability, and one can see that in her eyes within those photos. Although her dementia was diagnosed in her mid-70s and is in so many ways different from mine, maybe it is more similar than I wish to admit.

22nd May – London

I am really pleased to have been invited to join the Dementia Truth Inquiry. Consequently, today was a positive day for me, enabling me to come to terms better with what's been happening over the last few weeks. It was energising to throw myself into a new project, and one that looks so interesting, with two people who are so keen to positively support me with my engagement in it. I was invited by Nada to join this project at the Mental Health Foundation, and during the course of this I'll be supported by her and Sophie. This will provide me with much-needed and welcome continuity, which for me is the best therapy at this stage. The Truth Inquiry is designed to consider and investigate how truth should be used with people in the late stages of dementia, primarily in care homes, but much more broadly throughout society generally. Truth to me is fundamental. I always tell and seek the truth, in conversations, beliefs and philosophy, and I hope that I can bring something and in turn take something from this project.

Within the panel which I've been asked to serve on, there are two other people with dementia, two carers, the same number of former carers, and a wide range of professionals from various disciplines such as psychology, psychiatry and neurology. The Alzheimer's Society are also represented, alongside Innovations in Dementia and the Joseph Rowntree Foundation. Toby Williamson from the Mental Health Foundation and Dr Daphne Wallace, who also has dementia, co-chair the group. Today was really establishing what and how the project/inquiry will work and investigate alongside confirming the timescales required to achieve the Inquiry's key aims. Another positive feature for me with my dementia is that not only will the support be consistent throughout the project, but we will meet at the same venue, at the same times, and every two months, which will sustain my ability to engage without forgetting, which unfortunately is normally the case with projects which meet every 6 to 12 months.

23rd May – London

Travelled today to London, this time with Lewis supporting me, to Thomas More Square, the Alzheimer's Society offices close by Devon House. The Canterbury connection with the name of the venue struck me, as the head of St Thomas More is buried in a vault in St Dunstan's Church, Canterbury. This is the first time I've helped with staff appointment interviews with the Alzheimer's Society, and I understand it's quite a rarity for the society to engage with a person with dementia in this capacity.

Reflecting later today, I felt the process was mixed. We interviewed four candidates, and initially I wasn't given a question. I merely got the sense that me being there was a tokenistic gesture. Lewis wasn't allowed in the interview room, and had to go and occupy himself by talking to Janet Baylis in the library, doing some private study in there, and going out, I guess, to explore the area around Thomas More Square. All of that, I thought, was far from satisfactory. Although I had no support from Lewis, or anyone really, I did manage to grab the opportunity to ask a question, which the panel and subsequently I heard from the successful candidate was felt to be a key question. This was around exploring what made each candidate 'tick' as a person. The professionals on the panel can and should focus on the professional attributes of candidates; where people like me can best contribute is around how the candidates make us feel – could we engage with them if they were supporting or working with us as a person with dementia? What was really, really positive about the day was the person who we chose to offer the job. The four candidates were from a strong field. Three of them we interviewed in person, and the fourth person, Lisa, was interviewed via Skype as she was visiting family in America. She was amazing in the interview, and it was one of those rare occasions where the hair on the back of my neck stood up, and I sensed the panel all felt the same. She really blew us away with her answers and her personality, and the way she came over. Consequently, it was an easy decision at the end to be able to offer her the job. I look forward to working with Lisa in her capacity as the engagement and participation officer for London.

25th May – Canterbury

Having resisted joining Facebook for many years, today I decided to take the plunge and join. I did this because I sense the importance of it in maintaining social contact with people: those I still see, those I no longer see, and those I see currently who are going to leave my life and move to other areas, and may wish to keep in touch. Nick, my son-in-law who devised the 'envoy' title for me, helped set it up for me on my computer. I'm not going to go for hundreds of friends, like many people do, but will choose my friends carefully – people who really are true friends – and then share important things with them through occasional postings. I get a sense, with the dementia and life in general, of the importance of making and maintaining connections with others, and this could be another way of doing that. I hope so.

29th May – Canterbury

I felt privileged to have such a good attendance at the annual review of my envoy role at St Martin's Hospital. Supporting me were Jon Parsons, a director from the Mental Health Trust (KMPT); Janet Lloyd, who has been so encouraging, from the patient liaison service at KMPT; sterling allies in the students Alex, Sophie and Lewis; and the ever-loyal Reinhard. The meeting was really positive and I felt fully respected, valued and supported. I look forward to continuing next year in the role, albeit after July with different supporters, but maybe some of those will be able to maintain the excellent support given to me this year. For me this counterbalances to an extent the upset I increasingly feel around sensing that my world and my freedom within it is shrinking due to my dementia. I have many conflicts now inside my head, especially if I put it above the parapet to 'be shot at', which results in feeling exposed, lonely and a target. This in turn exaggerates my sense of guilt about having dementia and then down comes the fog. It is only because of the network of friends and family who try and help me that I am able to carry on.

2nd June – Canterbury

Today was the last appointment with Dr Beats at Gregory House, because she is retiring as a consultant psychiatrist, and she wasn't able to tell me who would be taking over with me. She did though put my mind at ease by saying that it would be someone who would be well able to continue monitoring my care. I do so hope that the new person and I can sort me out a care plan worthy of the name.

4th–6th June – Canterbury

Had a lovely few days with Hellen Riley, one of our Australian friends who's visiting us. One highlight was to walk in the warm June sunshine along the riverside from our home to the Parrot pub in Canterbury and back again. The walk and the conversation were lovely and much appreciated by Hellen. When we arrived home, with a glass of Aussie wine in our hands, as a Facebook devotee she encouraged and helped me to make better use of it, along with helping Rosemary master her new iPad.

9th June – Canterbury

Sophie came to my house today to work on her poster on the Forget Me Nots, which she is constructing for the Faculty of the Psychology of Older People (FPOP) conference in Shrewsbury. Reinhard had been trying quite hard to get me to attend and go with them to Shrewsbury, but I'm not sure this is right, and I have resisted it. I am not going to go, but through helping her with her poster, I get a sense of connection to the conference and those attending.

My files and notes are better than those at Gregory House on the Forget Me Nots, so she was able to access a lot of information which I'm told will be useful in constructing what she needs for an effective poster presentation.

14th June – Ramsgate

Today, Rosemary and I went to celebrate a friend's birthday. The friend is Tessa Reed, who is the chairman of the EKIDS group, and she invited us to join her to celebrate at her party. It was a very pleasant evening, and one highlight for me was to meet up after a gap of over 30 years with Angela Chandler, an ex-pupil from Littlebourne School. She looked at me, and I looked at her, and apparently she said, 'That looks like Mr Oliver!', followed by her coming over and having a chat. I'm so pleased that she had the courage to do so, because we spent a while chatting. Rosemary also remembered her because when I taught at Littlebourne Rosemary used to come in and help teach sewing with the children, and Angela was one of the children who participated in that. She was a lovely girl then, and she's a lovely woman now. I was also thrilled when she told me she had gone on to be a primary school teacher, and part of the reason for this, she said, was being taught by me, back in the early 1980s.

Coming away from the party, the one word that was ringing through my mind was 'reconnection'. It's so wonderful to have that opportunity, and such a privilege.

15th June – Rye

Rosemary and I took a complete break from dementia, and used our rail pass for a rare occasion to do a 'jolly'. We took the train from Canterbury down to Rye. The sun shone, and it was a lovely day. We had lunch at the Mermaid Inn, which is in the centre of Rye on a cobbled street. Another highlight was to browse around the antique shops and stalls, which are located by the quayside.

18th June – Canterbury

I was collected by a taxi today to go to Canterbury Christ Church University, where there is a recording studio operated by students and Radio Kent. The reason is that I have been asked to attend the BBC studio in London to record an interview with David Cameron, the Prime Minister, tomorrow. I refused because I have another meeting tomorrow, and I didn't want to cancel it. Clearly they wanted my involvement in the project, and arranged for me to be recorded in the studio as part of *You and Yours* on Radio 4. The interview was conducted by a really pleasant journalist named Winifred Robinson, who put my mind at ease and asked me questions about dementia. I think this is in light of an announcement to be made by the Prime Minister in the next few days. The idea is that they'll interview him, and edit the two of us together, before it is broadcast on Radio 4 in a few days' time.

19th June – Canterbury

My final meeting with the three amazing students who have given me such wonderful support this year. This was followed by the last writing workshop in the afternoon at the Beaney. It was a lovely sunny day, so we met on our patio and looked back over the year, discussing some of what we have done together. The conversation was fuelled by some juices that I had made, and we played a game of Guess What Was in the Juice. We also talked about the transition to the new students, and how we can best support that.

20th June – Canterbury

Party at Reinhard's with Rosemary to say thank you to the students. It was an enjoyable event, and though tinged with some sadness, tempered by looking forward to working on *Welcome to Our World* – a book that we're aiming to be published as a follow-up to the writing group. So it is very much a case of goodbye, but see you soon, rather than goodbye as an ending, which in my current state of mind with dementia helps me a lot.

24th June – London

Because there were no students available for today's Alzheimer's Society service user involvement workshop, I was supported by Angeliki, an assistant psychologist from St Martin's Hospital who I know through her support with the Forget Me Nots. She did the same as the students would do, and joined in by participating as if she was a member of Alzheimer's Society staff. It was a really good day.

This was the first of these workshops I am co-presenting with Lisa Bogue, on whose interview I helped with recently. Lisa, although shy and not experienced at presenting to and teaching an audience, was really very good, and keen to learn from the experience. I am sure she will be able to apply her really excellent personality to the role alongside growing professional skills.

28th June–5th July – Avignon, France

Holidays are so important to everyone for being restorative, energising and stimulating, and this was certainly the case for Rosemary and me in Avignon, during which we explored Provence. Whenever going on holiday, although it requires more planning and preparation, we do try to visit new places as well as returning like a boomerang to Adelaide. So often people with dementia either are advised not to travel, or feel themselves that they are not capable of travel. This certainly need not be the case. I am lucky that together Rosemary and I are good travellers who like the same sort of places and are willing to make compromises when needed.

We travelled using the Eurostar direct from Ashford to Avignon, which makes the journey so easy. Highlights of the holiday were the journey itself; the historic sites within walking distance of the hotel, which was conveniently located in the town centre of Avignon; then beyond Avignon we explored the region using public transport to take in the lavender and sunflower fields, which were at their best; and culturally the city of Orange with its substantial Roman buildings.

10th July – London

I travelled with Rosemary to the six-monthly executive committee meeting at the Royal College of Psychiatrists. After helping me to settle, Rosemary left to have lunch with our son Gareth in St Katharine Docks.

During the meeting I was sitting and talking with Noel Collins, who I had met previously and shared a platform with at conferences at the British Psychological Society. Noel is a very friendly Australian psychiatrist who is an advocate in involving people with dementia, so consequently, along with the encouragement of committee chair James Warner, I am beginning to feel more comfortable within this esteemed group.

15th July – Whitstable

As part of the follow-up element of the writing course, I have funding to support the five students in working with the eight writers over the summer period to produce work which can then be turned into the book *Welcome to Our World*. The students were allocated two writers each, generally speaking, and the student supporting me and Chris Norris is Sophie. Today, she and I went for a memory walk at Whitstable. The weather was glorious, and in a relaxed frame of mind we were able to talk about the writing and the book in general. By applying what I have learnt from the writing courses, today was basically walk, talk and write.

17th July – London

Another one of the service user training days with Lisa, who this time was more confident but just as lovely in her presentation skills, and I was well supported today by Sophie who, like her predecessors, engaged enthusiastically in the workshop activities.

19th July – Blean

This evening Rosemary and I went to Blean school for the first time in a considerable while to support John Davies, the caretaker, who is retiring. Although it was good to see old colleagues at his leaving party, I found the crowded hall and noisy band very difficult to cope with, so we left early.

23rd July – Windsor

Twice a year, the over-50s club from Shepherdswell organise a visit, and today's was to Windsor, which for us was very special because it enabled us not only to see the castle, but also to take time to meet up with our daughter and grandson in their new home which they have just moved into. Whilst the amount of time we could spend with them was all too brief, it was great to see them happily settled in their new home in Windsor.

24th July – London

The Truth Inquiry now is rolling forward and meets every two months. Today was my second panel meeting supported by Sophie. Having spent the first meeting generally talking about 'What is truth?' and establishing our thoughts and aims for the project, today we interviewed a number of witnesses who came to present their views on truth based upon their experience of dementia.

The first witness was a carer named Ming Ho whose mother has dementia. Ming was able to talk about her experience of living with her mother both before she had dementia and since, and then the continuation of their relationship now her mum is in a care home.

The second witness was Paul Baker, who comes from an organisation called Hearing Voices Network, and this was around how voices can be heard by people when in fact there are no actual voices. He explained the difference between reality and not-reality, and what strategies can be used to better support people experiencing this – for them the voices are truthfully heard.

A third person presenting was Professor Arlene Astell, who talked about truth and dementia from an academic point of view, and gave us thoughts around labelling and distress, and living in the here and now. She talked about how false realities can be a positive and also a negative from her perspective as a trained clinical psychologist.

It was a really interesting mix of witnesses speaking with us and we are beginning to ascertain and establish what vocabulary should be used in connection to discussing truth. Alongside the inquiry meeting the discussion on the train home with Sophie broadened my understanding of the subject and I am gaining a better understanding, especially regarding 'delusion', in the sense of being the person with dementia's understanding of reality. Fascinating stuff.

28th July – Canterbury

Tried to work on a photo album of my mother's photos, but couldn't manage it. It upset me too much. Again, part of this is seeing my mother as a well, vibrant, intelligent young woman. That was my mother, in her 30s and early 40s, and to witness her decline through first bipolar and then Alzheimer's filled me with such immense sadness. The emotional and cognitive scales tip heavily towards the former on days like this and the flood gates open, and I struggle to close them again. I've decided to park that task for the time being, and hopefully return to it later, because there are photos which I want to be able to treasure, and to keep in a way that they deserve, alongside making a similar book for James, because she thought the world of him.

29th July – Canterbury

What was a very pleasant meal today was interrupted by me not being well. We were at the Parrot pub in Canterbury, which has become one of our favourite places to go to. I was with Rosemary, her sister Barbara and Michael, our brother-in-law, and I had not been feeling too well during the course of the meal. When I got to the point of having the dessert, I really felt as if the whole room was revolving around, and I was going to faint. Apparently I went ashen white, and looked really ill. I *felt* really ill! The bar staff were notified, and water was brought over to try and help, but it did no good. I wasn't really aware of what was going on around me. A swift decision was made that an ambulance was required, so one was called, which arrived quickly. I was taken out to the ambulance and made comfortable. The paramedics took my blood pressure, which apparently had fallen to a worryingly low figure. After about 30 minutes I felt a little better and wanted to return to my meal and in-laws. I was told that I was not well enough to do so. After almost an hour I felt well enough to get up, and by now I felt embarrassed, and uncomfortable in the situation. My whole life now is feeling so abnormal at times and alien to me and this was yet another example of this. I wanted just to get back to normal, but was told I had to stay put. The blood pressure hadn't restored to normal, so the ambulance crew made the decision to take me to hospital. I was taken to Kent and Canterbury, thankfully, and not Ashford, where I was placed in a room whilst they monitored me.

Looking back at the timings of today's incident, the ambulance was called at 1.30, and I arrived at the hospital at 2.45; by 6.20, I was deemed well enough to be discharged, and Rosemary and I got a taxi home. I was totally drained and exhausted physically and emotionally. I will go into see Frances, the manager at the Parrot, this week and apologise as I do feel so embarrassed and guilty – an emotion I feel often now with my dementia but have not experienced with other health issues to this point.

4th August – Canterbury

Having recorded the BBC Radio 4 show *You and Yours* involving the interview a couple of months ago, that was broadcast with the Prime Minister, today we did a follow-up with the show to coincide with a meeting of the Welcome to Our World team (that's what we've become now as that's going to be the title for our book), which will be funded by an Alzheimer's Society Innovations Fund grant Janet Baylis and I have managed to secure. A number of writers, the five student supporters, plus Elizabeth Field; April Doyle; Katie Bennett, media officer from the Alzheimer's Society in London; and John, a producer and journalist from the BBC, recorded the interviews alongside a planning meeting. The planning meeting took place with Liz in her summer house, and we were each taken into her lounge by John to be interviewed for the radio programme which will be broadcast in a few days' time.

I was reminded, today, of an African saying that I picked up in a book recently: 'If you want to go fast, go alone. If you want to go far, go together.' I, and others in the project, really do sense that this is a 'together' project, that there is a team of 14 of us working with a shared purpose and a common goal, and challenging so many preconceived negative images. If we can pull this off, it will be great, and if we can produce a book written by eight people with dementia, supported by Liz, our wonderful teacher, and five incredible students, then that will be a really amazing achievement.

6th August – Whitstable

Today Alison Culverwell, the senior psychologist for the region, picked me up and drove me to Whitstable to speak to the East Kent Care Dementia Programme Board, who had not heard anyone with dementia speak to them before. It was rather like going with Reinhard a few years ago to speak to the Trust board. I can't remember what I said today, but I remember that I felt quite welcomed by the board, and I got the sense that members were genuinely interested in my words, so consequently I came away feeling positive.

12th August – Canterbury
Following a visit on 9th July by Ian Asquith to my home, today he came to say farewell because he is now going to begin his doctorate course in Sheffield. He wanted to talk about our ADI project, and to follow it up, and good intentions are that maybe we can return to it during the course of his doctorate. I didn't want to place any undue expectations upon him with this, and he goes with my very best wishes, and the hope that maybe, in the future, our paths will cross, because the dementia world isn't a large one.

13th August – Canterbury
Sophie came to my house today as a follow-up to our writing and walking session four weeks ago, and we carried on writing and working on two pieces which were unfinished. It appears that I and one other person are contributing more than anyone else to the book. There are a number of reasons for this, part of which revolves around the really good support that I am receiving, and the inspiration and enthusiasm that comes with that.

After the writing, Rosemary joined us, and the three of us listened to the 'Welcome to Our World' broadcast on *You and Yours*, a piece that was recorded at Liz's house nine days ago. I was pleased with the piece that John had done. All the interviews came over really well. The only negative, I thought, was that one person was excluded. They had used seven of the authors, and not the eighth person, which I thought was very sad. I would rather that they had cut the seven slightly, and made them seven slightly shorter pieces, in order that all eight could be included.

18th August – London
Back up to London for an IDEAL (Improving the Experience of Dementia and Enhancing Active Life) project meeting in Queen Square with Reinhard and Sophie. Before going to the meeting, Reinhard took Sophie and me around Bloomsbury, and was really keen to talk to us about the Bloomsbury set, which gave him the opportunity to share his knowledge. It was something I had heard of but didn't know much about, and I smiled

to myself that a German guy was able to teach two English people about something from within our own culture.

In the evening, having got cheaper tickets through the Alzheimer's Society, I was able to go to Wyndham's Theatre with Sophie supporting me to see Carey Mulligan and Bill Nighy in a play called *Skylight*, and afterwards we met Bill for a photo and his autograph.

22nd August – Canterbury

Apart from the days when I have felt well supported, I haven't been well for a little while now, I guess since the hospitalisation day. Life has been a real rollercoaster, so I decided to see my GP. I've been losing quite a bit of weight, and my weight now is down to around about 13 stone, whereas before, I was a comfortable 14 and a half. That was one concern. I'm also not hearing very well, or not absorbing what I'm hearing. My blood pressure, which I'm now monitoring, is quite volatile. Sometimes it is too high, sometimes it is too low. I seldom have headaches, but I'm having those now, and getting very upset over things.

I don't often go and see the GP, as my diary illustrates, but I do feel that today was quite helpful. He said that I'm clinically depressed because of my dementia, and that in itself was stark to hear. I said to him that I've been trusting my instincts for many years, but now they are deserting me, and I don't know how to handle that. He was encouraging in what he said. He tried to suggest antidepressants. My response did not surprise him, but the way I expressed it did. I said to him that 'If I am going to go down then I will do so with my eyes wide open.'

I left the surgery with a sense of relief that he now knows what I'm dealing with and the impact my dementia is having on me.

28th August – Canterbury

One positive aspect of Facebook at the moment is that the Motor Neurone Disease Association are organising something called the Ice Bucket Challenge, and everyone I know seems to be participating. Having been nominated by Reinhard, I am keen to be involved. Out of my cupboard, I got my Nottingham Forest shirt from when I went to Germany in 1979 to watch Nottingham Forest play in the European Cup Final. The German link was appreciated by us both.

Having poured ice over myself, filmed by Rosemary in our garden, I posted the piece on Facebook. Putting on that shirt did take me back, briefly, to when I was 22, and I still fit in it! I was then able to nominate Angeliki, Jean and John to soak themselves in freezing water.

This episode also inspired me to pick up my pen and write a piece using techniques taught to me by April in the writing course. She had given us the *starting line* and the instruction to write for five minutes; here is what came out of this:

'*There at the very back of the wardrobe I found...* Hidden amongst trousers, jackets and ties, most of which hung limply and dormant like the memories of a former life they evoke, something which meant much more to me. It was far more than a shirt, it was an episode from my life, seldom worn, even when new, and now constrained to sharing space with cluttered clothes. A shirt I bought aged twenty-three for a special occasion. A shirt to identify my allegiance and a connection which had stretched back to being a child aged seven. A unique shirt for a unique occasion. An occasion when we felt special, invincible, on top of the world. A special shirt for a special adventure, packed into an old, spartanly furnished train carriage heading off into the unknown. A shirt with an emblem, a reinforcement of attachment, a badge – as Stephen Crane would describe in his famous novel – it was a "red badge of courage". We all looked the same, although we were all different. Whilst most memories dim, flicker and then fade, the shirt allows these memories to shine as brightly as a rocket's glow, one which is transporting me back in time. Now once again I am twenty-two and not fifty-eight; now once again I can see the comet which so fleetingly came into view and lit the dark sky. Now I touch and thank the old shirt, fold it carefully and place it in a drawer where its status is much better suited, until next time...'

30th August – Faversham

We went over to see Melvyn and his wife Jan. For some time they had been trying to get us to come over and spend some time with them. Melvyn drove us to a country pub near Faversham Creek Rosemary and I had been to before, but some years ago. I think Jan really appreciated it as well, because she doesn't get out as much as she used to, and Melvyn enjoyed the company and was in good form. It was a sunny, memorable day for us all.

1st–2nd September – London

Nada invited us to attend and participate in a Joseph Rowntree event entitled Dementia Without Walls. This involved an overnight stay at the Royal Foundation of St Katharine, in Limehouse. The event's aim is to bring together people with dementia, carers and professionals from all around the country for two days with an evening in between to share experiences and thoughts around the Dementia Without Walls project. It's really interesting and inspiring to mix with people I'd heard of before, such as Agnes Houston, but have never met.

During the evening of the 1st September, the mood was lightened by a really entertaining piano recital within the complex which was very therapeutic and soothing.

4th September – London

As a change, a coach trip to London with the U3A to visit William Morris's house and Olympic Park. In the case of the latter, the last time Rosemary and I were there was prior to the Olympics, and the site was under construction. That was in 2010. Whilst we didn't attend the Olympics, for reasons I've already written in my diary, around not knowing whether I'd be well enough when the lottery for tickets became available, it was really good to be able to see the venues as they were used in the Olympics. We spent most of our visit admiring the velodrome, which was awe-inspiring.

The Olympic Park is picturesque, and it's good to see the buildings which were used as the Olympic Village being utilised for accommodation today for people living in this revitalised part of London.

7th September – Whitstable

Rosemary and I spent this morning with Amy Merritt and her husband Steve, along with their young daughter Rosie, at Whitstable Castle. This was the culmination of an exchange of emails between Amy and myself which came about through Amy hearing me on the *You and Yours* programme recently. She was a pupil of mine in the mid-1990s at Swalecliffe, and our paths had separated when she was 11, when I moved on to my first headship before she transferred to grammar school.

Now Amy is a young woman, and married with a family, and it was great to be able to reconnect, and to be able to share stories from her childhood. She was genuinely interested in knowing about how I had been, and what the intervening years had brought for me. Steve, very kindly, took Rosie off into the grounds of the castle and kept her entertained whilst Amy, Rosemary and I were able to talk.

11th September – London

One theme of the Truth Inquiry today was around some of the professionals revisiting a concept they introduced at the beginning of the project, which was around training colleagues to tell better professional lies. My viewpoint at the time remains the same, which is that I'd much rather the professional be trained to tell better truths. I have a real problem with people lying. I don't lie myself, and I don't expect other people to lie to me. I'd much rather people think truths, tell truths and share truths in a compassionate and person-centred way.

An example of this, as mentioned before in this diary, was with my mother, who when she was increasingly affected by Alzheimer's would ask where my dad was, and when he was coming to visit her. My answer would be, he wasn't coming today. This was perfectly true. The fact that he was never coming again, because he had died, was less important. If I had told her that, it would have reopened the grieving and the wounds that followed his death.

Similarly, my view on false environments and mock-ups of lounges and living rooms from people's former lives is changing. At first I thought this was a constructive idea, and would reconnect people back to their past. Now, through re-examining this in the Truth Inquiry, I am very unsure of its merits. It needs careful handling, which I don't always think care homes have the staff, time or expertise to do. I fear re-immersing someone in an environment which reflects something from 30 or 40 years ago, and then transfers them back to 2014, is very confusing and disorientating. They are likely, I feel, to wonder where people are who shared that space with them back 30 or 40 years ago, and of course many of them are no longer around.

The third aspect of the project, which by this time I'm questioning, is around the use of dolls, known as doll therapy. I accept this works for some people, because the doll can provide a sense of comfort, but many of those people, given dolls, take on the role of parent, and the doll becomes a real human being. Now I'm not sure about that.

We discuss all these issues in the project, and I'm able to talk through further with Sophie, who is supporting me on the project, going up to London and coming home. Without influencing me at all, she helps to clarify my thinking, feelings and memories of the project.

12th September – Canterbury

A Forget Me Nots meeting which marked the transition from last year's amazing student supporters to the new cohort. It also gave me the opportunity to update the whole group on progress regarding *Welcome to Our World*. To do this I attempted to read an extract from Jo Brand's wonderful foreword to our book. When I got to the phrase 'here is a book that shines a little light' I was overcome by the emotion and choked up. I couldn't complete the piece. Alex thankfully came to my rescue to help me out.

16th September – London

Reinhard, Chris Ryan from the Forget Me Nots and I attended the DAA meeting at the British Psychological Society headquarters in Tabernacle Street in London along with Charley, one of the former students from last year, who is happy along with Sophie to cover the summer before the new students start. At the meeting, I spoke alongside Chris Ryan about the Forget Me Nots, outlining what type of psychosocial support we require to allow us to live well with dementia. We also looked at the writing project, which both Chris and I had been involved with, and used the opportunity to platform what the project is achieving around challenging negative views of people with dementia.

We spoke about the book which will be called *Welcome to Our World*. A fitting title, we thought, and we gave them a flavour of the book without spoiling the 'cake'. There's a double pun here, because the icing on the cake was provided by Jo Brand, who at the moment is doing *The Great British Bake Off: An Extra Slice* on BBC TV, and has taken time out to write a splendid foreword to the book.

19th September – Margate

There are some days when the trauma of having dementia is more significant than others. Today was one such day. With support I went to visit Queen Elizabeth The Queen Mother Hospital, to observe a patients' drama therapy session for older adults led by a therapist named Katie and assisted by Sophie.

It brought to mind some personally troubling thoughts. First of all, it placed me back in the 1970s and early 1980s, when my mother was in a similar hospital, and was showing many of the behaviours that patients were displaying in this session. There was a lot of anxiety, a lot of expressions of depression, and a lot of behaviours that were quite difficult to observe. The way that Katie handled this was admirable, and the way Sophie supported her and the patients was genuinely compassionate, and reinforced my sense of respect towards her kindness because she was a rock to those patients.

I wonder what my mother would think if she saw me in this environment, and if she knew that I was dealing with dementia. All these thoughts and feelings were spinning inside my head as I left the hospital at the end.

22nd September – Canterbury

The Welcome to Our World project is significantly moving into its next phase with a final meeting of everyone at the Beaney, except for Lewis who was unable to attend. We discussed the project, and how it would move now into a book using the material the eight of us have written with the student supporters. We were joined by a photographer, and Andrew Bence, a writer from the Alzheimer's Society *Living with Dementia* magazine, alongside a KMPT Communications Team member. There was much excitement to accompany the news that the work was now with the publisher, and the second half of the meeting was devoted to planning for the book launch which is likely to take place in November.

24th September – Canterbury

Earlier in the year we held the annual meeting to discuss the future of my role as an envoy; today was a parallel meeting, held at my house, to discuss the future of the Forget Me Nots, and my and others' roles within the group. Attending today were Reinhard, Elizabeth and Angeliki, the local assistant psychologist. I've been feeling thin-skinned and vulnerable recently, creating greater strain on myself, and I feel the once positive experience of being in the Forget Me Nots has become an additional challenge through the attitudes of a few difficult members and my faltering confidence to co-chair.

It was a positive meeting, but a sense of friction, which I had detected from a few members of the group, was reflected in some of the points brought up by Reinhard and Elizabeth. We tried to consider how to address them together. We'll now have to see if those thoughts will work in action.

I think the emotions around Welcome to Our World and the book project, and lots of other things I don't understand, are contributing towards this, not just for myself but for others as well.

26th September – Canterbury

After the stresses elsewhere I do so enjoy talking to the occupational therapy students at Canterbury Christ Church University. It's a rare occasion for me to repeat an event from year to year, and whilst I update my presentation, fundamentally it remains the same, whereas most of my talks are written from a blank screen.

29th September – London

MSNAP (Memory Services National Accreditation Programme) conferences at the Royal College of Psychiatry are prestigious events attended by leading figures of the dementia world, including Alistair Burns, who I met for the first time. Rosemary, Reinhard and Chris Norris accompanied me, and we joined forces with Rachael Litherland at the event. I used in my talk today a piece I had written with Sophie and Liz Jennings's support around the day I saw the neurologist for the first time which resulted in the suggested diagnosis of dementia. I read the extract from *Welcome to Our World* to a silent auditorium. I sensed the piece was having a powerful impact. I felt energised by that, and reassured that its inclusion in *Welcome to Our World* will be a useful contribution to the book. Alongside this, it gave me an opportunity, with the audience, to provide an advance notice about the book, which seemed to generate a lot of interest.

30th September – Canterbury

I now acknowledge a transition in my student supporters from being alongside Lewis, Sophie and Alex, to a new group, and today the three for this year came to my house to meet with me. Their names are Jess, Ingrid and Laura. The idea, this year, is that the Forget Me Nots and the students will use a close buddy system, and it will be interesting to see how that works.

We had a really positive discussion. I focused upon them getting out of the placement what they put in, and already we have begun planning for the end, by seeing it as a ten-month project. They all seemed fairly shy, pleasant young people, not quite as confident, I would say, as last year's group. I'm sure we'll get on well together. I'm looking forward to getting to know them and working together.

6th October – London

Now that the Alzheimer's Society has split its research portfolio into two halves, I feel I am really getting into the care aspect of it, which is where I'm placing my energies. Today I attended a Research Network care panel meeting in London at Devon House, and was accompanied and supported by Ingrid.

This was the first time Ingrid had been up to London with me. She comes from London, so she knows the city well. As she became more confident, and more comfortable in the role, she really opened up and we had some engaging conversations which made for a good day for us both, primarily based upon her interest in the research.

8th October – Canterbury

A follow-up writing day, from 1st October, with Alex and Sophie, where we sat in my house and planned and wrote our presentations for forthcoming conferences, these being Alzheimer's Europe in Glasgow, which is this month, and the UK Dementia Congress in Brighton, set for November. The two subjects we are going to present are Welcome to Our World, which is with Alex, and the Forget Me Nots, which is with Sophie.

There has been generous support from the Friends of Mental Health in KMPT. Once again, what was clearly evident was the talent, commitment and support given both to me and to the projects from Alex and Sophie. They helped me enormously with the writing, including making suggestions around content. It really is a true example of co-production and co-thinking, and will, I'm sure, be a good example of co-presenting. Alongside that, they've both taken much of the pressure off me regarding the challenging administration linked to the conferences, particularly the one in Glasgow, which has been very complex.

Similarly with the travel, they helped with booking the train and the accommodation. I truly wish for harmony, unity and friendship within this project between the five of us – that's Alex, Sophie, Reinhard, Rosemary and myself.

13th October – London

Following on from the panel meeting last week, those projects which are likely to be funded were placed before the Care, Services and Public Health Grant Board at the Alzheimer's Society. Each member of the panel (there were 12 of us, 11 former carers and me) takes turns to represent the panel on the full board; today it was my turn.

The majority of members of the board are academics from universities around the country who have a particular specialism in dementia. They listened to the views of the four of us from the panel on three or four projects each, which made it manageable.

Most of the projects that the panel felt should be funded were agreed by the board. Their views and ours were, reassuringly, very similar. The next stage is for the society's trustees to consider the applications and recommendations before releasing any funding.

20th–23rd October – Glasgow

I am writing this diary entry in a Holiday Inn in Glasgow. Rosemary, Alex, Sophie and I made the immensely long train journey from Canterbury to Glasgow on the day before the Alzheimer's Europe conference started. Reinhard joined us at the hotel having flown up here, because he had another meeting to attend in London.

In our cases we have 95 copies of *Welcome to Our World* spread between us all. It will be interesting to see how many of these will sell. Already, on day one, we have sold half of them. Part of this was down to the presentation that Alex and I did, supported by our Forget Me Nots presentation which Sophie and I did, during which I was amazed to see that she had learned every word of the script. I could never do that, even before I had Alzheimer's.

During a keynote speech by Geoff Huggins, head of the Scottish National Dementia Strategy, in the main auditorium questions were invited. This gave me a platform (1) to ask him a question, (2) to comment favourably upon what he had been saying, and (3) to plug the book! At that point, I encouraged Alex and Sophie to stand up next to me and hold up the book.

Bit of a cheek, really, but I thought it would work, and it was justified by the number of people coming up to us to buy the book afterwards, thus raising money for the Alzheimer's Society. Amazingly, we sold 83 copies during the two-day conference.

27th October – Canterbury

A couple of weeks ago, I heard from Gregory House that my consultant replacement for Dr Beats will be Dr Richard Brown, and today was the first appointment I had with Richard. As I wrote when mine and Richard's paths crossed previously soon after being diagnosed, he is an ex-pupil of mine, and now I can tell people that I used to care for him, and now he cares for me.

In that context, he was interested to know how I was and how I've been. I wanted to use this as an opportunity to press him for the care plan that I am still awaiting. Whilst he was more positive towards this idea than Dr Beats, nothing was forthcoming today. Having said that, he feels that the time is now right to increase my dose of galantamine from 16 mg to 24 mg, which I believe is the maximum. He wrote a prescription for me, which I'll collect and start tomorrow.

I explained to him that, over the last three months or so, I've been experiencing a most difficult period, which is quite alien to me. I used to think I was bulletproof and armour plated. Now I'm sure I'm not. I described to him a tidal wave of tears, fears and anxieties around dementia and life in general. Even as a child Richard always had a serious nature, and his body language and tone of voice conveyed the serious way he saw my current situation. Hopefully help alongside the medication will be forthcoming.

31st October – West Middlesex

Ingrid accompanied me a couple of weeks ago to London, and today it was the turn of Jess. We went to West Middlesex Hospital to monitor the PREVENT project. This is the project that began just over a year ago when I was supported by Lewis. Now the project has moved to a state-of-the-art unit called CIDS (Cognitive Impairment and Dementia Service), which is a wing of the West Middlesex Hospital. The meeting lasted from approximately 12.30 until about 2.30. Professor Ritchie, the lead investigator for the project, proudly gave us both a tour of the new dementia unit, which was most impressive. The meeting finished earlier than I expected, giving

Jess and me the opportunity to get the train and underground to Devon House to meet Janet and Katie regarding the *Welcome to Our World* book, and to confirm arrangements for the imminent book launch.

3rd November – Canterbury

Sumita Chauhan, who contacted me recently regarding support for her PhD, visited me today. The subject for her PhD is digital arts and dementia. She is an artist who uses computer graphics and 3D structures to convey her creativity, and she wishes to find out more about people with dementia in order to run a project with them, which can then inform her PhD. Sumita was brought into my world by a phone call from my GP at the last Forget Me Nots meeting, which caught me completely off guard and totally surprised me, because he's never done that before. He told me that he had been at dinner with this lady, and they were talking about dementia, and her wish to find out more. His immediate thought was, 'I know who she needs to speak to. She needs to speak to Keith Oliver.' So he rang me to check if I was happy for my details to be released to her, which of course I was.

I enjoyed talking with Sumita and we had a very enlightening conversation. I didn't understand a lot of what she was trying to do by way of the technical aspects, and I suspect some of what I said around dementia passed her by. But between us, I think we found some middle ground which will be constructive.

4th November – Canterbury

Because I am searching for some deeper sense of support and peace, I attended with Rosemary a Spirituality and Dementia conference this afternoon at Canterbury Christ Church University. It failed to inspire me as its focus seemed superficial and centred on meditation and mindfulness rather than deeper spiritual thinking.

6th November – Canterbury

After weeks of preparation, tonight was the book launch of *Welcome to Our World* at Waterstones bookstore in Canterbury. The event went extremely well, due in part to the participants – the people with dementia, who are the writers, the student supporters, family and friends. Claire, the manager at Waterstones, has been an ally during the planning phase and was happy to provide refreshments for this evening's event. After the talks and readings approximately 70 books were sold, and we had an audience in excess of 80. Claire told me it was the biggest event the store had ever mounted.

Each writer was invited to choose a reading from their contributions. Many did, and those who felt unable to do so delegated this to the student who supported them. Finally, the students read pieces from their contribution to the book, which endorsed the idea of it being a team effort. Liz and I shared the Master of Ceremonies role, and the enjoyable event went really smoothly. Now the task is to promote the book and sell it in order to raise money for the Alzheimer's Society.

10th–12th November – Brighton

Following the Glasgow conference, this time Rosemary, Sophie, Alex, Lewis, myself and Reinhard travelled down to Brighton for the UK Dementia Congress (UKDC), partly to launch the book. On the evening of the first day, Rosemary and I went with Nada and Rachael Litherland to meet fellow activist Chris Roberts and his wife Jayne at a local pub. We had a really convivial conversation with them. I had heard about Chris but never met him. We established that beyond our link of having dementia, we also shared a link through having lived in Nottinghamshire, me as a youngster, him as a miner.

On the evening of 11th November, Rosemary, Alex and I were invited to the gala dinner by the Alzheimer's Society and joined their table. It was a really pleasant evening with lots of good food and wine and lively conversation, supplemented by a comedian who amused us all from the stage.

The UKDC is always a good event, and this is the second time I've attended it at Brighton, so both the hotel and the conference venue are more familiar to us.

15th November – London

I feel increasingly part of the Royal College of Psychiatrists executive committee meeting, to the point where they're asking me to do things for the committee. On this occasion, it's to write a piece on young onset dementia for their newsletter. Afterwards, I met up with Rosemary, and we went for a coffee with our son Gareth, which provided a very pleasant end to the day.

21st November – London

As part of the Alzheimer's Society Research Network, I attended a training session today with Jess, the student supporting me. It was extremely interesting to hear researchers talking about their projects, and to share networking with other people within the network. Jess is a very able supporter, and she and I are getting on very well in this role. I'm grateful to her for the support that she is able to offer by way of conversation on the train, and support during the meeting along with outward and return travel.

27th November – Chatham

Through contact with Alisoun Milne at Kent University, I was asked today to speak to social studies students at the Medway site. The talk went well, and I attended with Rosemary who drove me up there, but I do find the campus very difficult to navigate, and parking was a nightmare, which didn't put me in the best frame of mind when arriving to give the talk.

28th November – Truth Inquiry

Now Sophie needs to focus upon her final year of studies, this was the last event that she has committed to supporting me with. Coincidentally, Reinhard was amongst the people we interrogated today as part of gathering evidence for the project. Jess has eagerly offered to take over supporting me with this project, which I am pleased about. I am sure she will bring as much to it and take as much from the project as Sophie did.

1st December – Canterbury

As part of a project for the BBC, today I was filming at home with a camera that reporter Jim Reed had left for me when he came for the book launch three or four weeks ago.

Today, I filmed myself in the bathroom showing how I now try to remember to clean my teeth and shave, etc. This is by getting all the items out of the box, and as I use them, placing them back into the box so that at the end nothing remains on the unit. Later in the day Jess filmed the idea of me continuing with a hobby that I've had for years, which is stamp collecting. Rosemary has also filmed me at various locations, including Brighton. The idea is to make a video diary, which will then be used in the new year on the *Victoria Derbyshire* show, to coincide with the launch of the movie *Still Alice*, which focuses on young onset dementia. The programme concept is that three people who have differing experiences of young onset dementia will be filmed and included in the programme: Wendy Mitchell, who has not long been diagnosed, myself occupying the middle space, and Christopher Devas, who was diagnosed some years before me, being the person who has been living with dementia longest.

I have been thinking about the students, and when walking in Whitstable on my own whilst Rosemary was at art, I was reflecting on the three currently supporting me. Whilst I am comfortable with the support from two of them, I think I need to discuss this with Reinhard at the next opportunity.

2nd December – London

It's the time of year for the DAA annual event at Westminster Hall, and the DAA generously supported Rosemary and me to stay in London last night. This was the first time that we had been able to do this – usually we have to travel up on an early morning train. Not having to get an early train set us up in a good frame of mind, and allowed us to attend a scoping planning meeting before the main conference, with a small group of professionals, looking at the possibility of establishing a national Young Onset Network. This is a great idea which has my full support and I wish to be involved. In this positive mood, the main event which followed was really good.

4th December – Canterbury

Having been filmed by Rosemary and Jess over the past four weeks, today Jim Reed returned with professional equipment – cameras, lights, sound recording equipment – and filmed a detailed interview with me at home. What I remember, thinking back on it this evening, is his focus on the sense of frustration that I feel around living with dementia. He also asked me what I would remember about the day, to which I responded, 'Very little, except for how I was able to feel, which was well supported.' Rosemary, Jess and Ingrid were in the background offering me encouragement, which helped relax me a little and gave me a sense of companion-ship. Even an audience of three helped, before going out on TV with a bigger audience.

10th December – Canterbury

Because of the way my health has deteriorated over recent months, through Reinhard and Richard, I have been offered a course of therapy from Jane Roberts, a psychotherapist at St Martin's Hospital. Starting today we went over background issues, allowing Jane to get to know me and giving me a sense of what the therapy may seek to cover. I do really hope that this course of treatment will help me.

16th December – Canterbury

Yesterday I had an appointment with Richard Brown, and today I was able to receive the results of the blood tests, all of which proved negative for whatever he was considering. The symptoms continue, but the explanation is less clear.

17th December – Canterbury

Began a new international project led by Alistair Burns and coordinated by the International Consortium for Health Outcomes Measurement (ICHOM) involving people from around the world. Today's meeting was conducted by video conferencing. This is alien to me, so to enable me to access it, Rosemary joined me, and we were supported by Ingrid and Jess.

It was really stimulating, and the time that was chosen for the meeting was 1 p.m., which meant that people in South America and North America were able to participate, alongside people in Australasia. There were four or five people from around the world with dementia, including Kate Swaffer, and six professional academics.

Previously ICHOM have worked on cancers, and the aim is to construct a list of health outcomes which can then be used to help inform dementia care.

22nd December – Canterbury

Having seen Richard last week, I had an appointment with him again today at Gregory House. He wanted to see me, as I have been struggling lately. He also wanted to check that the maximum dose of galantamine was working, and not having any adverse side effects, alongside sharing the results of the blood tests. Beyond this, he wanted me to explain to him what impact I had felt from the first consultation therapy session with Jane Roberts.

I was able to say that it was quite favourable in the sense that we were simply getting to know each other, and there was certainly the sense that she was going to drill deeply into a number of issues over the forthcoming months. I emphasised with him the hope that this will help me.

30th December – Canterbury

Today, and on 23rd December, I had two appointments with Jane Roberts. One area she was interested to explore with me was around family and my background. I think what she was examining there was what impact my childhood and my youth had on me today. She was also interested to find out what life was like for me with dementia, and told me that although she had done lots of therapy work, and lots of work with people with dementia, she had never actually undertaken this particular programme of therapy with anyone before, so that there's an element of each of us learning as we go along.

We talked about truth, and about honesty, and the importance of applying that which is important during these sessions. I explained how I often feel threatened by what is happening to me, which I never did previously, and how now I feel constantly that I have to defend myself, which leads to me feeling isolated and vulnerable. She talked about separation, and the issues around separation that I had earlier in my life, and that maybe they are impacting upon me now. I'm not sure what she knows about me since I was diagnosed, either through conversations with her colleagues or through reading my notes. Time will tell how useful this will be.

31st December – Canterbury

Saw the GP. End of a very up and down year. Not only have there been more foggy days than experienced in 2011, 2012 or 2013, but the fog has been thicker and slower to lift. However, when it does, the sun usually emerges and shines brightly and with warmth upon me. I did try and convey some of this with my GP and told him some of my thinking when the toxic mix of dementia and depression combine, and how my sense of perspective and positivity become greatly challenged. I talked to him about my recognition that living with dementia is getting harder and I know it will get harder still. He listened, but again, beyond adding to my notes and shaking his head in response to my rejection of antidepressants, I guess there is nothing more he feels he can do.

Thoughts going through my mind at this time are about how professionals and professional friends will relate to me, or wish to know me as they do now. I have a real fear that I will be dumped by many of them when the going gets toughest for me, when I need this support and engagement most. Usually when I feel down I turn to music to help lift my spirits, not to jolly songs but to reflective lyrics such as those by Leonard Cohen, who I am listening to an awful lot at the moment. I love his use of metaphor in the powerful lyrics he writes, which in my view stand up to scrutiny as poetry.

What will 2015 bring forward? I do hope for as many highs and sunny days in 2015 but rather less low, thick foggy ones.

Sometime in 2014

Dear Alzheimer's

Well dementia, in the year since I last wrote to you, it is clear that you've won some rounds but I still feel like I'm still winning the bout. It is now over three years since our initial encounter, and damaged though I feel, the damage is repairable with love and support, thus enabling me to search and find positivity in the fog.

I acknowledge that the length of the periods of time during both day and night you are with me is increasing. Even when I try to relax in my armchair in the evening, I need to grasp a cushion for comfort, but this does work, and by the time I rise from my chair, your presence has diminished. What has alarmed me is that you have recruited your toxic cousin, depression, into your armoury. To combat this, I sense the need for those around me, that is, friends and family, to be as positive as possible. I recognise that my bad days are their bad days, and my good days are their good days. The reverse for both of us is also the case. Whilst understanding that I need care, what works best for me against you is to be surrounded by caring people, and with their support and love, I see you retreat.

Welcome to Our World certainly was a rollercoaster ride, and your presence was never far away. I recognise this in both myself and the other seven writers. The challenges we faced were fuelled by you, and it was only through Liz and the five students that we were able to defeat you. No one could have anticipated that eight people living with you would ever be able to write a book of this sort. We have.

My wish and my hope is that people will buy this book, read it, and be inspired by it, alongside raising money for the Alzheimer's Society, a charity whose mission is to defeat you.

Ideas for writing have come easier than I could have hoped, partly inspired by those supporting me. This is in contrast to speaking in conversation at times when I get stressed and muddled, and then you wrest the words from my tongue or cause me to 'jump in' and interrupt for fear of you whisking away what I wish to say. But you never wrench away my thinking and my spirit, nor will you.

Clinging to the flotsam and jetsam of my mind in mid-ocean, there is a parallel for me; I feel a great sense of freedom when swimming in the ocean, and I thank you that my swimming skills have improved enormously since you came to reside. Things that used to scare me now no longer do so. Unwittingly, you have given me courage, where you wished to bring fear.

Disrespectfully yours

Keith

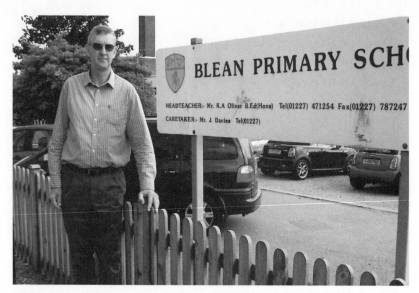

Keith outside Blean Primary School, Canterbury, around the time of his retirement (April 2011)

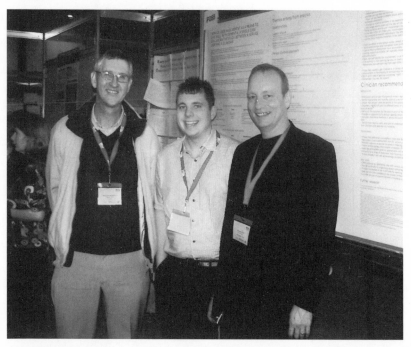

Keith, Reinhard Guss and Ian Asquith presenting a poster at the Alzheimer's Disease International conference, ExCeL centre, London (March 2012)

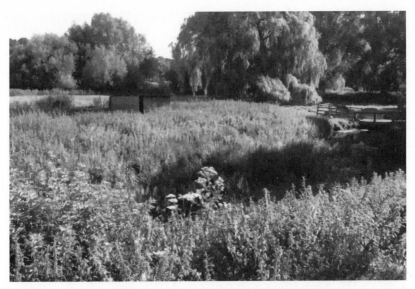

View over Hambrook Marshes and the River Stour (June 2014)

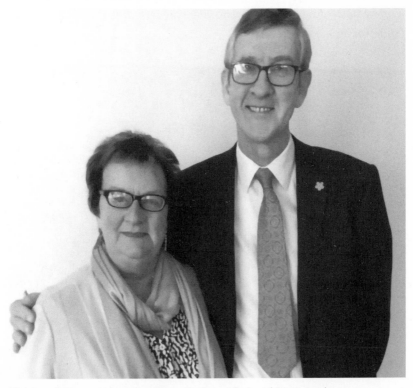

Keith and Rosemary ready to go to St James' Palace (April 2015)

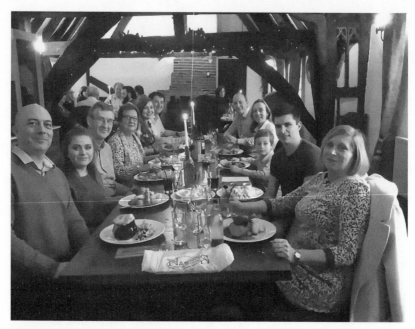

Keith's 60th birthday celebration with all his family at the Parrot pub, Canterbury (December 2015)

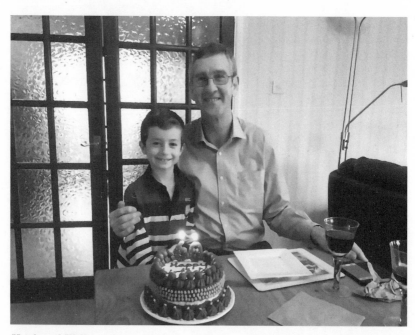

Keith and William, his grandson, on Keith's 60th birthday (December 2015)

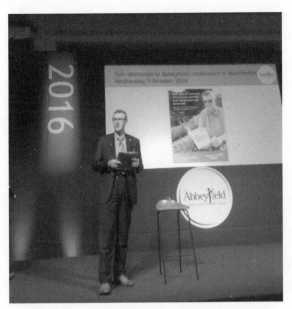

Keith speaking at the Hampton Court Flower Show (July 2016)

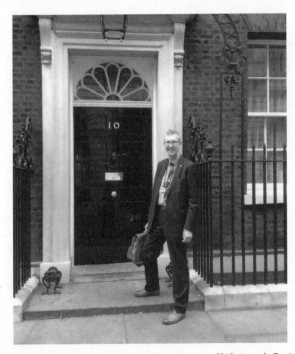

Keith outside No. 10 Downing Street going into an Alzheimer's Society event at the Chancellor of the Exchequer's residence (October 2016)

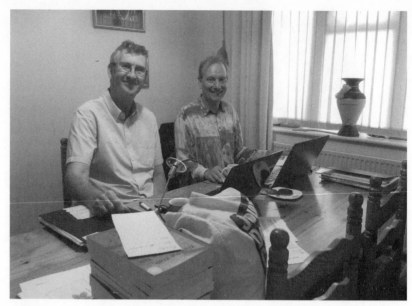

Keith and Reinhard working together to co-produce a talk for a conference (June 2017)

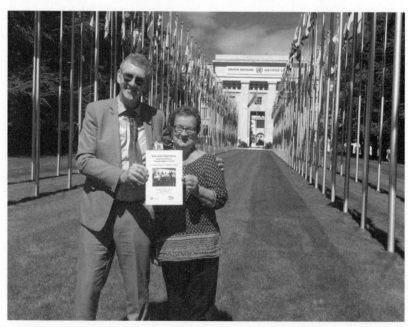

Keith and Rosemary at the UN CRPD in Geneva presenting the DEEP Think Tank document on the rights of people with dementia (August 2017)

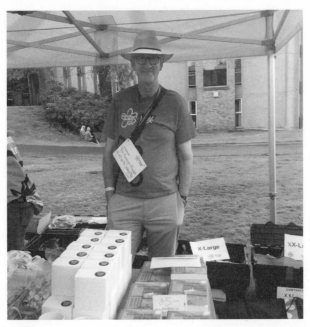

Keith at the Kent Memory Walk on behalf of the Alzheimer's Society at the University of Kent (September 2017)

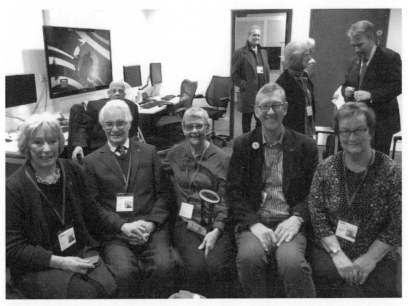

Veronica Devas, Christopher Devas, Wendy Mitchell, Keith and Rosemary in the BBC green room getting ready for the Victoria Derbyshire show (March 2018)

2015

—

'Therapies'

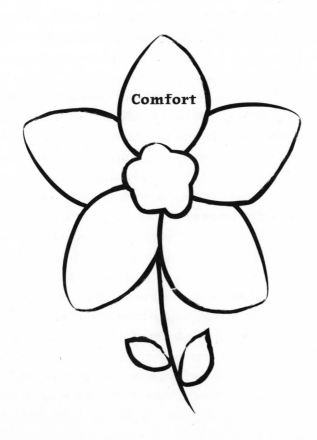

Comfort

2nd January – London

Yesterday I went to see the movie *Paddington* with Rosemary and really enjoyed it. Coincidentally, as tourists today we visited Borough Market, Covent Garden and Oxford Street, and saw statues which had been located around the city to celebrate the work of Michael Bond and this iconic character. Rosemary took a photograph of me, doffing my fedora next to a black and white statue of Paddington in Oxford Street doing precisely the same thing.

Whilst we will often tag on a relaxed fun element to close our days in London, today was a rare experience for us of being in London with no dementia meeting commitment.

5th January – Canterbury

After the Christmas break, I feel refreshed and raring to go, and the first dementia-related activity for me involved meeting with Jess and Ingrid, the two psychology placement students supporting me this year, who came to my house for a couple of hours of planning and writing with me. Last year I was able to lean upon Sophie, Alex and Lewis, and they in many ways became rocks for me to lean on and take strength from. This has positives but also risks, which I am mindful of with the two supporters this year. Able and willing though they are, I need to be vigilant to their needs as well as my own. I feel the end of 2014 and start of 2015 is something of a watershed for me as I seek to continue through being engaged, active and supported to find ways of living as well as I can with what dementia throws at me.

6th January – Canterbury

As part of my desire to find out more about life story work, and to explore how it can be used in the earlier stages of dementia, following on from the Welcome to Our World experience, I met today with Laura from Kent County Council, part of whose role is to explore how life story work can be utilised in community projects. Laura is lovely and enthusiastic, and I enjoy meeting with her. This is the second or third time we've met, usually tagged on to a workshop or a talk I'm giving to a group of professionals.

I think that life story work has a really important part to play before people arrive in care homes, rather than just reserving it until that point in their dementia pathway when others close to the person often write the life story document for them as the dementia is more advanced.

9th January – Canterbury

After a good week, today was the monthly Forget Me Nots meeting, and it reinforced the difficulties I am facing within the group and within my role as co-chair, alongside Reinhard and Elizabeth. I feel I am attracting a lot of flak and negative feeling from two or three members of the group, and that's what I dwell upon rather than the more positive approaches and feedback that I get from the other 15 members of the group. Because of my dementia I am now thin-skinned and find the difficult atmosphere at these meetings really immensely challenging. In fact, I find any difficult situation now extremely demanding and draining mentally, emotionally and physically. Alongside this, there seems to have been an increase in the number of emails coming in my direction connected to the group and my role in it. The agenda is hard to manage because there are so many items. I'm being leant on, I feel, from all directions, and losing sleep over this. Maybe it's time now to consider my future in the role, which is so disappointing as the first two years of the group were on the whole very positive.

12th January – Canterbury

Julia Burton-Jones from Dementia Pathfinders visited me today to discuss the YODEL project and my involvement with the Pathfinders. It's always lovely to meet and chat with her, and she's such a kind and thoughtful person; the project's focus on young onset dementia is an added attraction. Our discussion was, as always, fruitful and engaging, and we talked around issues connected to young onset dementia, what it is like to live with, and what my views are for professionals to better support those who have young onset. The outcome of this conversation will be recorded in a booklet.

13th January – Canterbury

Another intense hour-long therapy session with Jane where we focused upon my challenges in interacting with others and how this can at times be uplifting but at others immensely difficult, and is another example of the emotional/cognitive imbalance I now experience. I don't feel confident to talk about some issues and concerns, but I did mention to her about photographing on my mobile phone the Samaritans sign displayed on the bridge over the busy A2 near my house. She endorsed this move by saying that it showed I was trying to take some control over the fog and my emotions. I may well not use the number but it is there in case I do want to.

14th January – Canterbury

Following the immense success of *Welcome to Our World* I phoned Carly Turnham at the University of Kent regarding the psychology students who supported us throughout the project. I wanted Carly, an administrator within the School of Psychology, to know how amazing those five students were in that piece of work, and maybe to broadcast that fact within the School of Psychology. She thought this was a really interesting idea to explore, and offered to write a piece which will be included in the school's psychology newsletter. She asked me to send her a photograph of the group, which I'll do tomorrow.

A couple of days ago, I received an advance copy of a DVD from the British Film Institute (BFI), via the Alzheimer's Society, including all the BAFTA-nominated films for this year. The film they want me to focus upon is *Still Alice*, which tells the story of a young American woman (in her early 50s) who is experiencing dementia. I read and loved the book, and this will be a good opportunity to watch the film.

The Alzheimer's Society and the BFI want me to provide some feedback on the movie, and rather than do it on my own, tonight I'm having some friends round, including psychologists Reinhard and Elizabeth, plus students Jess, Charley and Lewis, and we'll watch the movie and give them feedback using a pro forma I have devised for this evening.

15th January – Canterbury

Following on from a really enjoyable evening watching and discussing the *Still Alice* movie – Charley's comment stuck out for me: 'Good film but not as good as working with real people who have dementia.' Chris Norris, Carolina and I, plus the student supporters, attended and spoke at a post-diagnostic meeting as part of the East Kent Transformation Group at St Martin's Hospital with the commissioners, led by Linda Caldwell. During the meeting we explored how the current provision works at the memory clinic in Canterbury for those with dementia, and how post-diagnostic support can be improved to support people beyond the diagnosis. I was a little overwhelmed by the packed agenda with only 10 to 15 minutes per item allowed.

16th January – Canterbury

I had an email today from Daren Kerle, who is the Kent community librarian for this area, to inform me that the library service in Kent have recently purchased 34 copies of *Welcome to Our World*, and will place them across the county in various libraries over the next week or two. I'm really humbled by this vote of confidence by Daren and Kent Libraries, and hope that readers gain as much as we did from reading the book.

20th January – London

Continuing the work with the Truth Inquiry, today I attended with Jess, and it's great that she's got into this project just as much as Sophie did before her. Today the expert witnesses were largely from the world of academia. We had Professor Lisa Bortoletti from the European Research Council who explained her views on truth in the late stages of dementia, and also Professor Dawn Brooker from Worcester University, who gave a really enlightened talk about her work within the university and beyond in working with people with dementia and how truth impacts upon that. Toby, the co-chair of the Inquiry, brought to the table a paper which is based upon some qualitative survey responses which have been drawn from people living with dementia who expressed their views on truth around a certain number of questions, included in which are confusion, hallucinations and delusions, alongside how professionals can best treat people with dementia as truthfully as possible.

22nd January – Canterbury

Following on from the evening spent watching *Still Alice* a week or so ago, today I had a phone call from Tony Seymour from *The Guardian*, which had been set up by Katie Bennett, media officer at the Alzheimer's Society. We discussed the movie and what life is like for me living with young onset dementia. I look forward to reading the article in the newspaper when it's published shortly.

24th January – Canterbury

I went on YouTube today, and was amazed to see that the film *Keith Oliver's Story* has now passed 10,000 views and seems to be attracting about 155 per week. I am staggered by this as I never expected anything like this when Mycal, Rosemary and I made the film in 2012 for Kent County Council and it was placed on YouTube in April 2013.

25th January–1st March – South Australia

Our annual trip to Adelaide. I feel like a 'boomerang' returning each year to visit dear friends and recharge the batteries in an environment where we feel safe, happy and secure, as well as warmed by the Aussie sunshine away from the depths of winter. It is as much the people – their humour, hospitality and warmth, which is every bit as energising as the Aussie sunshine – which draws us back.

After last year's diversionary trip from Adelaide to Port Lincoln, this time we flew out to Kangaroo Island. We had been on the island before with Alan and Glenys Brokenshire, but this year our time with them was spent in Adelaide and we felt confident enough to venture off alone. Speaking of Alan, we love going swimming, with him at the beautiful white sandy beach close to their home. The sea along the Gulf of St Vincent, which stretches along the coast around Adelaide, is so crystal clear and multi-coloured, ranging from rich shades of turquoise through to vibrant ultramarine, all of which contrasts so distinctly with the purest blue sky one could imagine. I feel so liberated when swimming, and despite our constant vigilance in the water for sharks and other nasties, aided by the hourly fly-over by the shark-spotting plane, I feel a sense of release from what dementia confronts me with. As I recently wrote in an email to a friend, swimming with the sharks, strolling with the snakes and sitting with the spiders is easy compared to living with dementia when the fog descends.

This trip has also given me time and space to think about my future, both within the Forget Me Nots and beyond. I feel a great allegiance to the group as a whole and to individuals within it – both professionals and members with dementia – but I also question whether I can sustain my present role for much longer.

3rd March – Canterbury

Jane Roberts was keen to see me for a therapy session soon after my return from Australia and to discuss how my mental health had been during the holiday. I was able to reassure her of the positive aspects of the trip.

When I got home I was thrilled to have received in the post a copy of the novel *Still Alice* from the Alzheimer's Society, personally signed to me by Julianne Moore, the Hollywood actress who was fabulous in the title role in the movie. This helped to compensate for having to decline an invitation to the premiere in London due to being in Australia.

Whilst away in Australia we, as always, recorded *Coronation Street*, which has left us with 25 episodes to watch! The only problem this year is that the recorder has jumbled them up out of sequence for some strange reason. However, it won't matter too much to me as I cannot remember the previous episode anyway!

4th March – Canterbury

Through the commissioners, the Forget Me Nots were invited to speak at a range of workshops with GP staff, and today it was my turn to speak with a group of about 15 receptionists from the local area. I spoke throughout alongside Anne, and later Mark, both of whom are fellow Forget Me Nots, and was led by Tanya Clover, who is being commissioned to coordinate this piece of work. I always enjoy co-presenting with Tanya, and today was certainly one of those lovely occasions.

I thought this was an important group to reach, and their understanding and awareness around dementia was raised by what Anne and I said to them, although I'm not totally confident of the impact and the positive difference it will make when they return to work in their surgeries. I was interested to note that there was no one from my GP's surgery in attendance today. Hopefully they'll go to another one of the sessions that are planned across the area over the next week or two.

5th March – Barham

I attended the funeral of Stephen Hambrook, who was ex-chairman of governors at Blean school, and who was a very loyal and reliable ally to me during my time working at Blean. He was the classic critical friend within the governors, and helped put into place with me a number of improvements to the school, especially around the building stock. Whilst less interested and comfortable with the curriculum side of the school, Stephen was really a great go-to for advice and support around buildings and finance matters. He was ex-military, and had served all around the world, particularly in the Falklands where, as a member of the Royal Engineers, he was involved in mine and bomb disposal work which resulted in an incident where he lost a leg due to an explosion.

9th March – Canterbury

The idea of a teleconference involving people contributing from all around the world was something which, previously, I would have walked away from. But with the support of Rosemary, Jess and Ingrid, this morning I am now more involved in this project coordinated by ICHOM.

Following the teleconference we were joined by Reinhard and Elizabeth for a Forget Me Nots planning meeting, where I announced my resignation as co-chair, outlining the reasons for this. Some were surprised, others less so. I'd given a lot of thought to this over recent weeks, and during our holiday in Australia, using the space and ability to sit down and reflect without distraction, it became clear to me that this was the right course of action to take.

I will announce it formally to the group at the next meeting on 13th March. Now I've shared this with Rosemary, the students, Reinhard and Elizabeth, I feel more confident in going public to the Forget Me Nots. It feels like a weight has been lifted off my shoulders. Rosemary asked me if I'm sorry about this, and my answer is no.

10th March – Canterbury

I was able at my therapy session today with Jane to discuss at length about the thinking around my resignation as co-chair of the Forget Me Nots, and having her listen attentively has proved helpful.

After seeing Jane, I went into Canterbury to collect the Welcome to Our World paperweights I'd commissioned. The designs look really good: engraved images of a book and the name of the person alongside the name of the project, Welcome to Our World. They're lovely mementoes for people to keep, and I hope that people like them. Each of the contributing writers will get one, plus the five students, Liz and Janet Baylis. I'd saved approximately £200 from the grant to allow for something of this sort to take place at the end, the two options being a memento or a party. The paperweight seems much more fitting, particularly since we celebrated the project at the book launch back in November 2014.

12th March – Canterbury

Liz and I met with the manager of the Curzon cinema in Canterbury today to discuss whether the Curzon would be happy to provide us with an affordable venue for the movie project that we're looking to launch later this year. The manager was really keen and interested, and it does appear to be an excellent venue. At the end of the meeting, when pushing her on the cost of hiring the space, she offered us a special charity rate, but this was still too expensive and I don't think, despite the attractions, that the Curzon is going to work for us.

Due to a number of reasons, not least of which the challenges that dementia presents me with in managing to keep on top of commitments and the changes each week at Wincheap School in location and timetabling of the children, I have decided the time is right to call it a day on going in and hearing the children read, before I feel I am letting them down. It has been a real privilege and pleasure to have this opportunity and it has enabled me to gradually break away from my former life in primary schools with the children and staff. As a lovely gesture the teachers had a collection and today gave me a lovely standard rose named 'Top Marks', which they chose partly for its name which the accompanying card described as 100 per cent fitting. Another inspiring example of the positive impact plants and flowers have on my life, and very much in keeping with the 'Kitwood flower'. There are so many kind people out there who I am so fortunate to know.

13th March – Canterbury

Today I announced formally to the Forget Me Nots my resignation as co-chair. Similarly to the professionals and the students, some members were surprised and some less so. It resulted in a discussion around resilience, and I made the point to one lady that I am now much more thin-skinned and cannot cope with some of the vitriolic comments that have come from her and one or two others. Consistent with her manner was her response that I should be more thick-skinned. Most people seemed sad and disappointed that I am resigning but one or two, I suspect, were quite pleased. The discussion I had with fellow envoy Chris Norris and Reinhard earlier around Chris taking on the role proved fruitful, as Chris agreed that he'd take on the role for a year to see how it goes, thus giving some degree of succession planning. I'll give Chris every support I possibly can.

17th March – Canterbury

Following on from the Forget Me Nots meeting last week, today Reinhard, Elizabeth, Chris and I, supported for note taking by the assistant psychologist from St Martin's, Angeliki, met at my house to discuss the transition of co-chairing from me to Chris, and what that will involve.

19th March – London

After the difficulties around the Forget Me Nots recently, it was a breath of fresh air today to travel to Devon House with Ingrid's support to be involved in one of my favourite days, which is the Alzheimer's Society service user training day, led by Lisa and me. As always on these days, which I have now done a number of, it was a really positive group of people who enthusiastically participated in our workshop. Ingrid, shy and reserved though she is, did engage very positively during the day, including being delegated to report back on behalf of her group on one aspect of the workshop. The day closed with some really pleasant conversation between us on the journey back to Canterbury.

24th March – Canterbury

Psychotherapy appointments with Jane Roberts are now coming thick and fast. Jane now schedules them for every week or two, because that's what she feels is needed and could prove helpful to me. One area she led me through today was around endings in relationships, which she likened to grieving. A while ago I would not have seen it this way, but now I can see that there is something in that.

25th March – London

Today was another really good day at the Truth Inquiry, once again with Jess's support. When we arrived at the meeting, we were able to spend some time in private conversation with Rachel Thompson, who had agreed to meet with me to discuss life story work, which allowed me to draw from her experience and opinions of this initiative and intervention. As this is an area of interest to Jess, she participated in this meeting as well, which will hopefully inform her own professional development.

Included in today's meeting, chaired by Professor Graham Stokes and Dr Daphne Wallace, was a presentation by Penny Garner from the Contented Dementia Trust; she spoke at length about the Trust, the book *Contented Dementia* by Oliver James, and the project it is based upon, called SPECAL (special early care for Alzheimer's). I have read the book twice and her presentation confirmed my overall negative views on this work. Whilst there are merits in advice not to question people with dementia, to learn from the person with dementia as the expert on their disability and to always agree with what they say and never interrupt, in reality at times these are unrealistic and put an enormous pressure on those who love and help care for us. I also found the fact that Penny failed to mention the word 'truth' once in her presentation rather disconcerting.

26th March – London

Rosemary and I had been invited to an important event coordinated by Steve Milton and Toby Williamson around dementia and human rights. A number of professional groups are seeking to align those of us with dementia with the human rights lobby, primarily through disability groups, and today was a starting point for this. I found it an interesting day, hearing various views around dementia and disability, with the keynote talks given by Peter Ashley and myself. Peter is very well placed to do that given his experience and levels of disability. Alongside this we had some speakers from the rights movement who don't have dementia, but have a range of other physical disabilities, and it was good to hear them speak about their experience and how maybe we can draw from that and utilise it as we move this campaign forward. For my ten-minute slot I focused upon Tom Kitwood and tried to outline what I saw as the key rights of people affected by dementia, and came up with these:

- The right to be treated with respect and love (I refer to professional love as shown in the flower in my talks) by those close to me – family, friends, professionals.
- The right to an accurate and sensitively delivered diagnosis, not to be seen as a statistic!
- The right to have one's wishes, views and cultural, spiritual and ethical beliefs respected.
- The right to be heard, listened to – *and* responded to.

- The right to psychosocial interventions/therapies, both post-diagnosis and pre-confirmed diagnosis, which are appropriate, engaging and helpful to me as an individual. There are cliff-edge moments when the fog descends and results in the malignancy. I just thought about that word. If it was malignancy connected to cancer then heaps of resources get allocated – rightly, but why not when connected to dementia?

- The right to medication for those with dementias that may respond positively, and the right to expect conscientious monitoring of this medication and any timely adjustments. NICE says that these should be available – wrong! It should be *will* be available.

- The right to quality information about one's own dementia and the services available to us through both signposting and encouragement. I would wish to see life story work brought more into the early/mid-stages of the condition, at a time when it is more useful and helpful to people, which takes better account of their ability to be involved in its construction and use. My mother's document, to the best of my knowledge, remained unused in the care home manager's filing cabinet. Crumpled and under-valued.

- The right to consistent and sustained professional support (the model of a care worker used by the charity Young Dementia UK (YDUK) is a useful one to examine) similar to the Admiral Nurse, which in some areas provides outstanding support for carers.

- The right of association – joining with others who share one's experience and desire to do something useful is very important, hence the importance of initiatives such as the Dementia Engagement and Empowerment Project. Our Forget Me Nots group in East Kent is one of over 50 groups linked into this across the country.

- The right to a care plan worthy of the name which draws together a partnership of professional and patient/service user and explains clearly what is in place to support the flower and diminish the malignancy.

- The right to be cared for by staff who are treated, trained and paid as professionals – so often people working with folk who have dementia are poorly treated themselves, low skilled and underpaid. No wonder that places such as care homes cause such fear in the minds of many.

- The right to travel – contrary to the advice of my neurologist to cancel our forthcoming trip to Australia when I was initially diagnosed with dementia, with support from Rosemary, Meet and Assist as secured by the travel agent and appropriate insurance in place, my right to travel is maintained.
- The right to laugh, to enjoy life through stimulating activities, which might be creative – music, arts, writing. Read Jo Brand's lovely foreword to *Welcome to Our World*, which reinforces this.

28th March – Canterbury

Having read and loved the book *The Boy in the Striped Pyjamas*, today I was disappointed that it was such a foggy day, which got in the way of my enjoyment of seeing the story performed as a play at the Marlowe Theatre. The book, by John Boyne, is a classic which I'll never tire of reading and re-reading. I enjoyed the film version, although not quite as much as the book.

Sitting on my own, my engagement with the play was very much affected by the fog that descended upon me, making me very anxious during the performance. Feeling agitated, I nearly left halfway through, but stayed because of my attachment to the story. I recognise that although I have only been to the theatre a few times on my own in my life, the thought of doing so without Rosemary or a friend is now beyond me emotionally. Also, reflecting now a few hours afterwards, I'm saddened by having little recall of the play, other than how I felt during it.

29th March – Canterbury

Fortunately this evening I felt much better, and coincidentally again attended the Marlowe, this time with Rosemary, to see a performance entitled *The Simon and Garfunkel Story* – great music, well performed by a duo who looked and sounded very much like the real thing. The guy performing as Paul Simon was a talented musician, and he captured Paul Simon's voice. The singer playing Art Garfunkel had the pose, the height, the hair and, most importantly, that amazing Art Garfunkel voice which really came into its own during his rendition of 'Bridge Over Troubled Water'. Although Rosemary and I saw Paul Simon in concert in 1991, I never saw this amazing duo, but I feel this comes close.

1st April – Canterbury

Nada visited me again today to discuss the IDEAL project. This time there were no mishaps in the taxi; last time she'd brought Rosemary and me some flowers which had leaked water in the taxi, and there was quite a laugh and a joke with the taxi driver about that when she got out.

During our discussion we talked in depth about the IDEAL project, which is seeking to recruit and research the views of about 1500 people with a diagnosis of dementia, and as close to that figure as possible for carers, then to repeat this over a period of five years in analysing attempts to live as well as is possible with dementia. The project is coordinated from Exeter University. My role is as an advisor, with the 'expert by experience' label.

8th April – London

At the BBC TV centre today for recording the *Victoria Derbyshire* TV show live. This followed on from making the video diary supported by Rosemary, Jess, Jim Reed, the BBC reporter on the programme, and Katie Bennett from the Alzheimer's Society. I really enjoyed this project.

At the TV centre, we met Wendy Mitchell for the first time, who as a participant is telling her story of a relatively recent diagnosis. I'm the person in the middle, and Christopher and Veronica Devas are telling the story as a couple for whom the diagnosis was a longer time ago. We were joined in the studio interviews by Joy and Tony Watson, who spoke as a couple, although they weren't involved in the video element of the story. I looked at my hands during the showing of the films and they were sweaty and clammy, which illustrates the impact the films had on me. Victoria Derbyshire was lovely and interested in what we all had to say, and this was coupled with some extensive, enlightening footage from our three video diaries. She professionally and compassionately put us all at ease.

Rosemary was with me in the studio, although not in front of the camera. She remained behind the camera with Katie Bennett, and was joined during the filming by Carol Kirkwood. It made Rosemary's day to have been able to spend time talking with Carol, the *BBC Breakfast* weather presenter.

13th April – London

The general election is now in full swing, with considerable discussion around the NHS, part of which I'm pleased to say has focused upon dementia care.

Through the DAA today, a pre-election hustings was organised in London, and I was invited to attend and ask a question on behalf of the DAA. Chris Norris and two of the placement students – Jess and Ellie – came with us. Standing in front of the invited audience were Jeremy Hunt, representing the Conservative Party, a Labour peer and a Liberal Democrat representative, to whom questions on dementia were asked. The event was noted and recorded by Jess and Ellie, and as we were leaving, this point was shared with Sarah Tilsed who helps coordinate the DAA. Sarah asked if Jess and Ellie would share their notes with her, which could then form part of the official record of the event. I was delighted, because I think both Jess and Ellie are diligent and conscientious, and this would give them a boost in what they're doing within their placement.

15th April – London

A year ago, Rosemary and I attended the Alzheimer's Society People's Award at St James's Palace as guests. This time the invitation was somewhat different, because today I am there as a nominee for an award entitled 'Realising Potential'. During citations in the ceremony, it was mentioned that my nomination was particularly unusual, because it was the first time someone with dementia had been thus nominated. Consequently, I didn't expect to win the award, and was absolutely astonished when my name was read out as the award winner. Again, the event was a lovely day in the sunshine – both outside and inside my head. Afterwards, Rosemary and I were able to spend time talking with Richard Madeley who was MC for the day.

Leaving the Palace, the sun was still shining, so we strolled through St James's Park. Alongside the brightly coloured tulips in full bloom, Rosemary took photos of me proudly holding the trophy I had received earlier.

21st April – Whitstable and Canterbury

As part of my morning walk along the beach at Whitstable, whilst Rosemary did art, I called in to see Jocelyne for a coffee.

The afternoon was rather less relaxed, with an intense psychotherapy session with Jane Roberts at St Martin's Hospital. I'm not sure whether it's my state of mind or the session itself, but I did find it particularly challenging today. The most challenging part of it is the elements which I term as being 'deadly silences', when I look at Jane and Jane looks at me, and nothing is said for what seems like forever, but is actually probably only a few moments and certainly no more than a minute. I find silence very difficult to handle at any time, but especially within the therapy sessions.

25th April – Herne Bay

This year's EKIDS annual trip was to Herne Bay for the Young Onset group to enjoy a game of crazy golf and a fish and chip lunch, both of which were great fun.

28th April–6th May – Cornwall

We're so lucky to have such amazing Australian friends in Julie, Paul, Wayne and Jan, especially when they are keen to come over to England from time to time. At present they're over here visiting and were keen for us to join them on a break in Cornwall, based in a cottage in Polperro.

Throughout this trip we hired a minibus which enabled us all to comfortably see the sights of the county, with Paul enjoying driver duties. During the visit we called into Port Isaac, where we'd been a few years before with Julie and Paul, and once again saw some of the sights connected to the *Doc Martin* drama. In addition we visited Looe and Fowey, and went down a fascinating tin mine near Penzance. What struck us all was the similarities between Cornwall and parts of South Australia by way of the coastline, the beaches and the industrial heritage connected to tin and copper mining which drew many Cornish folk to depart for a new life working in the South Australian mines in the nineteenth century.

6th–8th May – Herefordshire

Following our stay in Cornwall, Jan and Wayne departed and Rosemary, Paul, Julie and myself headed up to South Wales and Herefordshire. Over two days we saw a part of the country that Rosemary and I had never explored before, and which we enjoyed, including the beauty of the Black Mountains and some historic Welsh castles. Lots of laughs, lots of drinks and lots more good memories.

11th–15th May – Staffordshire

After a couple of days' break back home in Canterbury for Rosemary and me to recharge our batteries, we rejoined Julie and Paul, this time in Staffordshire, where we took a canal barge through the Potteries into the Staffordshire countryside for a relaxing, entertaining mini-break. Once away from the industrial archaeology, the rolling, soft countryside of Staffordshire was a delight to see from our canal barge, which was surprisingly spacious and comfortable. I didn't know that I'd be able to stand up inside it, thinking I might spend four days bending over. In fact it was very luxurious and well equipped, which made for an even more enjoyable time. Paul managed the steering and the boat, whilst Rosemary, Julie and I tended to devote our energies to handling the locks and being on 'bar duty'.

19th May – Canterbury

Psychotherapy appointment with Jane Roberts. I put a lot into these sessions and come away feeling drained physically, mentally and emotionally.

21st May – Canterbury

Having enjoyed Mark Haddon's book, today with Rosemary I went to see the theatrical version of *The Curious Incident of the Dog in the Night Time*. Because I felt better and more relaxed in myself, I liked the play as much as the classic book.

26th May – Canterbury

It doesn't seem a year ago since our last annual meeting to discuss the envoy role at St Martin's Hospital. Again this year I was supported by Reinhard, and Janet Lloyd and Jon Parsons from KMPT, plus Ingrid and Jess, the two students helping me since September last year. We were also joined this year by Chris Norris, who wants to find out more about the envoy role, and Christina Shaw, KMPT's director of communications, who kindly came down from Maidstone to record the meeting in writing for the Trust.

The meeting was very constructive and we discussed together reflections on the past year – the successes and the challenges. For me the challenges were largely around the Forget Me Nots chairing role and relationships in the world outside of my home. We also covered successes, including Welcome to Our World, and some of the activities outside of Kent that I've been doing in my envoy role.

The envoy role, though, can be quite lonely and isolating, as I've experienced at times, so I had a flash of inspiration which gladly proved positive in nominating on the spot Chris Norris to share the role of KMPT dementia envoy with me, and I was delighted when, shocked though he was, Chris accepted. I'm sure he'll be a great ally and a great credit to the role for a long time to come.

28th May – Canterbury

Jocelyne Kenny, who is getting close to completing her thesis on service user involvement in the world of dementia for her doctorate, visited me at home today to talk through her project and to seek my views on aspects of it before it is completed. Once we had finished talking about this, we were able to spend a little while in the garden sharing our love of plants and gardening.

1st June – Canterbury

Following an earlier meeting to discuss the IDEAL project, Nada and I again met at my house to look at writing an article for the *Journal of Dementia Care* on Welcome to Our World. Joining us today was Alex, the idea being that Alex and I will write the piece together and Nada will support and facilitate it.

4th June – London

We are now in the midst of trying to train as many Alzheimer's Society staff as possible in service user involvement, and Lisa and I have really got this off to a fine art. I love these days and I really enjoy working with Lisa, and feel privileged to see her confidence growing in her role of trainer. Today I was supported by Ellie, one of the students.

This evening is the first episode of the TV documentary series *Dementiaville*, being aired on Channel 4. Before moving into the world of care homes, the first programme introduced viewers to the main families involved, and through David Sheard, the expert advisor to the families, an approach to living with dementia was outlined and explored.

7th–8th June – Oxford

Rosemary and I had a lovely two days in Oxford, staying at Keble College within the confines of the university, after an invitation from Toby Williamson to speak about living with dementia from a personal perspective to a group of academics and researchers involved in a project that Toby is working on.

On the Sunday when we arrived soon after lunch, the sun was shining – it was a beautiful day – and we enjoyed the relaxed environment of the Keble College quadrangle and admired the superb architecture of the university before venturing out, walking into the city to enjoy a couple of hours as tourists. I've not seen Oxford in this way before, only passing by it or through it, so it was lovely to do this.

I had teased Rosemary about my experience of being a student in the 1970s and sharing washrooms and toilets; she need not have worried as, a bit like on jumbo jets, we turned left for business class (staff) rather than right for economy (student) rooms.

Having relaxed yesterday I really was focused and able to contribute positively to the project, focusing upon co-production and service user and provider relationships by examining elements such as principles, process, purpose and impact, all of which I felt comfortable outlining from my viewpoint and then discussing with the academics present.

9th June – Canterbury

As it is only seven days since my last appointment with Jane Roberts, I am not sure how much progress we are making. Whilst I feel that weekly psychotherapy, although well intentioned, is too intense for me at times, I am reminded of Professor Alistair Burns's statement that therapy only works when it is being paid for. Whilst I don't pay money for mine, I pay with myself, so hopefully this payment of mine will enable it to be effective.

12th June – London

Jess and I travelled to the Mental Health Foundation for another Truth Inquiry meeting. Today's meeting was different in the sense that its purpose was to bring together people affected by dementia with the support of Nada Savitch and Toby Williamson, without the academics who sit on the inquiry panel. We spent a lengthy time discussing what our views on truth are, alongside our thoughts gained from previous meetings when we've sat and listened to the perspectives of professional experts whom we've questioned. Now it was our opportunity to spend two or three hours discussing in depth what we feel truth means to us.

I recognise and applaud Toby and Nada's strategy because the Inquiry has gathered a lot of information over the period of the project, and whilst I have always felt encouraged to comment at previous meetings of the inquiry panel, today was a much more service user-led debate.

On the train home Jess surprised me somewhat by saying that the time she had spent with me was the best part of the placement for her. I am so pleased that she has risen to and embraced the challenges presented before her, and hope that she will go on after her studies to be an asset to any team serving the needs of people with dementia.

16th June – London

Reinhard, Rosemary and I attended a Young Dementia Network meeting today, where the Young Onset Dementia workstream on awareness and understanding is beginning to establish itself by getting to grips with the work around raising awareness and understanding amongst various organisations and professions around young onset dementia.

After the meeting, Rosemary and I went to the Houses of Parliament where we were taken to a committee room for a discussion with Channel 4 representatives about the launch of their documentary series *Dementiaville*. I was encouraged to say how positive the experience of being involved in the project over a lengthy period of time had been, and what the background to my involvement was. I have really enjoyed being involved; my only criticism of the project is that I really do not like the title, *Dementiaville*. It sounds like a place where people with dementia are 'plonked'! I'd expressed that previously in emails to Channel 4, and in meetings with the producer, but clearly that was one battle I simply couldn't win. They took the comment in good faith, but made the point that it was eye-catching and would appeal to a younger audience.

19th June – Canterbury

Ingrid and I met at my house to discuss her placement project, which is on the Forget Me Nots and the use of Twitter to promote the work of the group. I was happy to do this for Ingrid, but most of my comments were, I have to say, at best lukewarm around the use of Twitter. I personally don't like it. I find it much more difficult to control than Facebook, and I'm not interested in registering on Twitter or, indeed, using it. I also recognise some of the risks and benefits of social media, and the challenges to mental health it can promote. Having said that, I understand that it can be useful in careful hands, and I will be passively interested in what she and her successor who picks this up when her placement finishes do with it in connection to the Forget Me Nots.

23rd June – Canterbury

I love sitting in the sunshine having a cup of tea on our patio, and today whilst doing this I heard via email the amazing news that Alex, Sophie, Lewis, Jen and Charley all achieved first class honours degrees in their psychology studies at university. Great news and richly deserved.

1st July – Canterbury

Today was the hottest July day on record, with the thermometer reaching 36.7 degrees Celsius. Rosemary and I noticed the car thermometer peaking at 40 degrees in Morrisons car park. It reminds us both of the hottest day ever recorded, 10th August 2003, when the mercury in Faversham peaked at 38.6 and we had friends visiting from Crewe who as gifts had brought chocolates with them on the train!

The other significant event of today was going into Canterbury after hearing the children read for the final time at Wincheap, for an initial meeting with Eric Harmer. This has been set up with the support of Jen Holland to see if Eric can support me through his ministry within the Evangelical Church. I have been thinking a lot recently about whether seeking spiritual support will help me, and now I have the opportunity to try it; although nervous, I am keen to explore this.

2nd July – London

Rosemary and I attended a meeting at the Comic Relief headquarters on the Albert Embankment in London for a project entitled Dementia Words Matter, coordinated by DEEP. After the meeting we had a meal and went to see the Carole King story, entitled *Beautiful*, in the West End. I got the tickets for Rosemary and me to celebrate her birthday.

6th July – London

I'd been invited with Rosemary's support to attend an all-party parliamentary meeting at the House of Commons, focusing on arts and dementia. We were both interested to hear how different projects are being viewed by parliamentarians as being useful to support people living with dementia. Before the meeting, we took a diversion down to Devon House where we met a number of staff there who I now regard as friends – Gaynor, Jane, Sarah, Katie, Andrew and Janet.

7th July – Whitstable and Canterbury

Rosemary and I enjoyed a morning tea at Jocelyne's to celebrate her daughter Imogen's first birthday. This set me up positively for another appointment in the afternoon at St Martin's Hospital with Jane Roberts.

8th July – Canterbury

Winifred Robinson, presenter on BBC Radio 4's *You and Yours*, has specifically asked for me to be involved in a recording today for a broadcast linking up with Alistair Burns, in the Salford studio. The breaking story involves a new drug which is likely to be launched very soon, and which hopefully won't be another 'false dawn' and will be useful in treating Alzheimer's.

9th July – Canterbury

Went out this evening for a drink locally with Reinhard, where we talked about how I had been recently. I recognise how fortunate I am to be able to do this.

10th July – Canterbury

Following on from the *You and Yours* programme a year ago, which involved the conversation with the Prime Minister, David Cameron, the highlight of which was reconnecting with Amy Merritt, today Rosemary and I met with Amy for coffee in Canterbury. It was a lovely hour we spent chatting, and followed up a similar coffee and chat we'd had at Whitstable Castle last September. Reconnections have always meant something to me; now, due to my dementia, they seem to mean much more.

12th July – Canterbury

Still on an emotional theme, music is so important to me, and has been since I was a child. My early memories are of my mother listening to the radio, and my father playing records on a gramophone. As I moved into teenage years, I developed my own musical taste, and part of that was the Moody Blues, so this evening it was great to be able to go to the Marlowe and see and hear one of my heroes, Justin Heywood, performing. I was thrilled that Rosemary enjoyed the show as well. The songs and the voice remain as good as ever.

13th July – London
I spoke at the English launch of the BPS Faculty of the Psychology of Older People Early Stage Dementia Papers alongside Reinhard and Chris Norris; the subject for the talk was the importance of service user involvement alongside the growth of the DEEP network as evidenced through the Forget Me Nots. Reinhard had generously planned for us to have a substantial amount of time in a very packed programme with eminent psychologists speaking. This gave me ample opportunities to outline my views based on real experience of pre-diagnostic counselling and consent, cognitive assessment, communicating a diagnosis, post-diagnostic support and psychosocial treatments before handing over to Chris to talk about our group's involvement in the publications we were present to help launch.

15th July – London
When I feel well, I feel comfortable within the confines of the Royal College of Psychiatrists, but at times I find that forum very hard to engage, which breeds uncertainty in myself. Today was one of the better days, and I took along with me a copy of James Warner and Nori Graham's immensely helpful book *Understanding Alzheimer's Disease and Other Dementias* for them both to sign, as they are both members of the Royal College's executive committee.

21st, 28th, 29th July – Canterbury
Two more intense appointments with Jane Roberts followed by a one-hour appointment with my consultant, Dr Richard Brown, to examine how I am feeling at present. He is keen to prescribe additional medication to deal with my growing anxiety and low mood, but I am still resisting this as I feel it is positive social interaction, care and support that will see me through back into the sun.

24th July – London
Following on from earlier meetings with Nada to discuss the IDEAL project, I now feel that it is moving forward, and today we established a service user

group which we have named 'ALWAYS' – Action on Living Well: Asking You. This group has nine members, some of us with a diagnosis, some of us caring for people or former carers, and the idea is that we will provide the IDEAL team with knowledge and insight from our lived experiences which they can utilise over and above the 1500 people who are participants in the project. Today I was supported by Alex, and despite it being a very wet day we stayed on afterwards to meet with a writer called Lore Windemuth, who is working with Professor Ruth Bartlett from Southampton University on a research paper entitled 'Social Suffering and Dementia'. They want me to be a co-author of the paper with them. Today Lore interviewed me to ascertain my views on several aspects around the subject. I think at the moment I'm well placed to talk about it because the notion of social suffering is very much part and parcel of many of my days – rather to the surprise, I think, of both Alex and Nada who sat in and listened to the interview. The mask was removed and the barriers came down, revealing how on the many current foggy days I do find it harder to live up to the expression 'living well with dementia', and find this on those days to be a burden rather than an incentive.

Following on from this, on the return train journey Alex and I talked in depth about some of the issues I am struggling with at present. Her maturity and honesty mixed with empathy and compassion belies her youthful 21 years, and her wise counsel provided me with some 'missing pieces in the jigsaw'. My only frustration with this is that Alex and I are now unlikely to have much time in the future to talk along these lines as she moves from university into work, and I fear I will not remember what we have spoken about beyond the issues.

4th August – London

Through Claire Thorpe at the Alzheimer's Society, I was invited today with Rosemary's support to speak at the M2M Inspiration Academy. This is a group of largely young creative business people from private commerce who meet once a month and invite an external speaker to engage and inspire them in their life and their work.

Being the Inspiration Academy, I decided that the talk I would write would explore what I considered the word 'inspiration' to be and what the concept of inspiration means for me, and how so often it's a term that is bandied around without really total justification in its use. Sometimes people will refer to me as inspirational, and I'm not at all convinced that that is an accurate portrayal of what I am and what I do. The talk went really well, and I was told that I was inspirational to this group, but time will tell as to what impact it has in their life beyond today, both at work and beyond.

Every six months, I along with 11 carers and former carers attend an Alzheimer's Society Research Network panel meeting at Devon House; today I am doing so with Rosemary. We discussed a range of applications for money to support projects involved in care and wellbeing. After the meeting, I met with Jane Cotton and Katie Bennett, who'd asked me to speak with them about an opportunity to talk on *Newsnight* on the BBC, which I've declined because it is too late in the evening. I tend to 'sundown' and am not too good after 7 p.m.

5th and 18th August – Canterbury

Two more psychotherapy appointments close together with Jane Roberts. The sessions continue to explore my attitudes towards myself (largely negative), towards others (largely positive) and towards dementia (largely combative). I know that Jane is trying to get me to open up and it is easier for me to do so when talking positively about other people – I suspect I have always been like this – and now she is trying to get me to focus more on myself. My combative approach to dementia is being used constructively, although at first she seemed to want to talk about anger, to which I said I am not an angry person, never have been; I have seen too much anger in my life and work amongst others, and my role has usually been as a 'peacemaker'. Browsing in Waterstones last week I was attracted by *The Forgiveness Project* by Marina Cantacuzino which will, I am sure, fit in with what Jane is trying to get me to talk through around me being hard on myself.

6th August – Canterbury

The Alzheimer's Society invited me to attend a volunteer event at Canterbury Cathedral today, and I really enjoyed sitting in the audience, watching and listening, rather than needing to speak. Today's service user speaking was Lorraine Brown, from Medway. Lorraine did a very good talk about her life both before and after a diagnosis of dementia.

17th August – Canterbury

A sad day for those of who knew the great Richard Taylor from Houston, Texas, who recently very sadly lost his fight, not with dementia but with cancer. Our dear mutual friend, Kate Swaffer, organised an online tribute to Richard and asked if I would contribute, which I was honoured and delighted to do.

Richard was the first person I turned to for advice when seeking with Reinhard and Elizabeth to establish the Forget Me Nots, and it was good advice which I followed to the letter. When I met Richard at ADI in London in 2012 we immediately hit it off, and he was pleased to express this when signing a copy of his book, *Alzheimer's from the Inside Out*, which I had just purchased. He wrote: 'To Keith, we are kindred spirits. It is my honour to meet you. Best wishes on your journey. Thank you for making a friend of me. Richard.' I shall treasure this book and the memory and hope that I along with others can try to take inspiration from his eloquence, humility and drive. So long dear friend, you will be missed.

19th August – Canterbury

This time, rather than me doing the interview on my own, Rosemary came with me to the BBC studio at Canterbury Christ Church University where I was interviewed for BBC Radio Kent as part of a phone-in on dementia for the Julia George morning show. Julia was very pleasant and interested in hearing my story and asked me questions alongside talking to me. She did though make a comment at the end about me not seeming or sounding like I've got dementia; well of course, I've heard that many times before, and I replied to her on air simply the words 'Thank you'. I didn't want to argue with her, I didn't want to take issue with it or debate it further. It seemed to me the most appropriate words to respond to her stereotypical comment and to draw the interview to a close.

20th August – London

The idea of the service user involvement workshops being taken around the country is a very real one, and whilst it would be lovely to have the capacity and ability to be able to do that, I certainly realise that this is not going to be an option for me, so today the compromise position from the Alzheimer's Society was to film me at Devon House. They will then use that film around the provinces to help train staff who cannot get to London for the face-to-face workshops.

25th August – London

The DAA board meetings always have packed and stimulating agendas, and I now feel more comfortable in the eminent company of those who share a place on the board with me. Reinhard and I always spend time on the train journey there discussing the content of the agenda, and he is always very supportive during the meeting in helping me to engage in the discussion.

26th August – Canterbury

It was lovely today to welcome my cousin Jane and her husband Ian to our house for a meal and then to go with them into Canterbury to show them around the cathedral. This allowed me to connect back to my former self, taking schoolchildren and Australian students with Julie Reece on tours of the magnificent building and exploring its history.

28th August – Canterbury

Both yesterday and today were foggy days, and this culminated in me having a fall near the tumble dryer in our laundry at home when I hit my head, inflicting a cut on the top of my head.

Although on some very foggy days I do use a stick, this is the first fall I've had for some time. The fall shook me psychologically and knocked my confidence as much as it hurt my head.

31st August – Canterbury

The fog continues, and today I attended with Rosemary a party I had been looking forward to at the home of our friends Adrian Taylor ('Tats') and Anne Hobbs. I didn't feel connected during the day, and worried about going. Once there I continued to feel unwell and was disorientated; there were too many people, too much noise and too many distractions, and even people who I'd known for a number of years I didn't recognise.

1st September – Canterbury

I always feel a little sad when the last lily flower fades and dies as happened today, though my spirits were lifted by Eric's kind gift of a new Bible, given to me at our monthly meeting.

4th September – Canterbury

I'm beginning to feel a bit better now, and today I had a meeting at Café Solo with Liz, Rosemary and Frances James, who works at Kent University. She is taking on the role of helping us to recruit students for the films project. Frances is someone I have known since she was a child, because I taught her in the 1990s, although like many of these former pupils, our paths diverged when she was 11, not to reunite until over 20 years later.

We began to plan the project, which will be around showing people with dementia and carers a series of six modern films over a 12-week period in a local venue, and for the people then to discuss the films afterwards. One would liken it a little to a book club, but instead of using books, we're using films. Early discussions with the Alzheimer's Society suggest that they would be comfortable in funding this as a part of their dementia-friendly cinema initiative.

8th September – Canterbury

The appointment today with Jane Roberts focused upon looking forward to a transition, as Jane is about to retire and is very kindly helping to facilitate a handover from her onto someone else who will be able to support me beyond the next session. We both agree that there is a need for a continuation of some form of support and therapy.

9th September – London

Following the filming of me for the Alzheimer's Society service user training, today was thankfully a continuation of the face-to-face workshops with Lisa. Today I was supported by Lewis, who has recently secured an assistant psychologist post locally and is still able and willing to do certain events with me, despite the fact that he completed his placement 14 months ago. This is because last year's students, Jess and Ingrid, have ended their placement, and the new incoming students don't start until next week.

15th September – Canterbury

I really have been looking forward to meeting the new cohort of students. In the group there are five students on placement who I am likely to work with. This year we're not allocating students to Forget Me Nots as buddies, because last year it worked well for some students and people with dementia, but not so well for others. In my case, having Jess and Ingrid was a real treat and a totally positive experience, but that experience wasn't shared by all students and all Forget Me Nots. Now we have decided that the five students will work from a pool, and whoever from the Forget Me Nots, including me, needs support will contact the five students and see who can fulfil that piece of work. This seems fairer in the sense that more of the students will get an opportunity to support the work I do in London and beyond.

I was joined by Chris Norris in talking to the students. Giving Chris this opportunity now that he is also an envoy was a new idea.

Final psychotherapy session with Jane Roberts, and now she's handing me over to Yvette Kusel, the clinical psychologist from Folkestone. Although some of it has been 'tough therapy', I have appreciated Jane's professionalism in helping me try and deal better with what dementia and life generally are 'throwing at me' and I feel in a better place because of this.

16th September – London

I was asked to be a guest with Rosemary at the Dementia Friends Awards at Trinity House. It was a lovely event with a three-course meal and a range of awards being given out to people who richly deserve them for their work connected to the Dementia Friends initiative.

On each table there was a goody bag for each person, and within that goody bag was a copy of *Welcome to Our World*, which was lovely. It gave a boost to the project and allowed me to speak about it in the after-dinner speaker role and then sign the copies that were given to nominees.

22nd September – London

The focus for today's quarterly DAA meeting hosted by the Royal College of Nursing was around keeping people with dementia safe. My attendance was supported by Alex and Reinhard.

It was an interesting day, and whilst most of the focus was on physical safety and technology, there were elements of discussion connected to mental and emotional safety. From my perspective I would prefer that being developed more fully.

24th September – Canterbury
Rosemary, Liz and I attended a constructive meeting at the Gulbenkian cinema, where we met the manager to explore if the Gulbenkian could be a venue for the movie project. The manager there formerly worked at Stirling University; consequently she is very keen to be able to take some of her experience from there into Canterbury to support people with dementia. That is one of the positives.

The venue is superb, and she is willing to give us the flexibility we require with a choice of programming – we can choose the films, which is something that both the Curzon and the Odeon were unable to do for us. The negative side is that the theatre is occupied for student lectures during the week, so the only free time we can have access to it is at weekends, and that won't work for us as we want to run the project on a Thursday morning.

The other negative is that it is over two miles outside of the city, and whilst on a bus route, it isn't as easy to get to as something centrally located, and car parking can sometimes be an issue there.

25th September – Canterbury
Time flies and it's my annual talk to Year 3 occupational therapy students at Canterbury Christ Church University with the support of Pat Chung.

30th September – Wimbledon
Rosemary and I travelled up to Wimbledon to participate in the launch of the Dementia Pathfinders document on young onset dementia. On the stage speaking during the day, alongside myself, were Peter Watson from a carer perspective, Dominique Kent outlining the work of the Good Care Group in supporting young onset people to live independently in their own home, and Jeremy Isaacs, who spoke from a medical perspective.

2nd October – London
Through an invitation sent out by Nada, Chris Norris, Rosemary, myself and Nicki, a student from this year's group, attended the trade union UNISON's annual conference. We were joined there by Dianne Campbell, who is another person with young onset dementia. Chris, Dianne and myself spoke passionately about dementia to what was a very different audience of trade union delegates. I also focused upon the care element of their work, because

most of them work in public service within the care industry, in hospitals and homes, and I thanked them sincerely for what they are doing. I also raised the challenge of what can be done to make things even better for those they're caring for and for them professionally.

6th October – London

For the first time, the Alzheimer's Society invited someone with dementia to speak at their annual general meeting, and they chose me. Rosemary came and sat with me during the meeting. My keynote address was about my experience of why, how, where and when I have been involved in engagement with the society. I wrote my talk for and directed it at the trustees, staff and volunteers present. After speaking I was fascinated to hear the annual report from the society, and to gain some insight into the accounts and the inner workings of the society that were shared at the AGM.

8th October – London

Within the national network Rosemary and I feel very comfortable as part of the Young Onset Dementia workstream. We are now beginning to identify groups which we feel would benefit from greater awareness and understanding of young onset dementia, and are narrowing our enormous list down to a manageable size, hoping at the next meeting to move forward with one starting group to focus upon. My personal feelings are that this should be the GPs, because they have a key role to play in both securing an accurate diagnosis and then constructively assisting a person to receive whatever suitable post-diagnostic support may be available.

12th October – Ashford

With Tricia Fincher's support, I delivered a talk at the Kent County Council library in Ashford to library and Gateway staff. There was also a Dementia Friends session led by Tracey Schneider which I participated in. I can't use the same strategy I used to use with Mycal Miller of being planted in the audience, because my profile is now too well known.

15th October – Canterbury

An initial getting-to-know-you therapy session with clinical psychologist Yvette Kusel. She explained her role and I told her something about myself, although I suspect she knew some of this previously from her colleagues and from what is written on my records. The first approach she is going to take will involve cognitive behavioural therapy (CBT).

21st October – Canterbury

Liz, Rosemary and I met at St Mary Bredin Church with an administrator as we've been told that we may be able to use a room for our movie project free of charge, and this would get round many of the barriers and hurdles that we are confronting by using one of the city's cinemas.

Connected to watching modern films, Rosemary and I went last week to the cinema to see the film *Suffragette*, at the Gulbenkian theatre, which we both enjoyed.

22nd October – London

Through Jane Cotton, I was invited to give a talk to the fundraising team at the Alzheimer's Society. I recognised and acknowledged the importance of their work both to the society and to those of us who access their services.

29th October – Canterbury

Two appointments today at St Martin's back to back, first with Yvette Kusel and later with Richard Brown. I do feel that both Yvette and Richard understand me, and in a focused but not uncomfortable time with each of them I can discuss my fears and anxieties around the challenges that dementia is presenting to me. With Yvette we are drawing the CBT to a close and she tells me we will move on to compassion-focused therapy which she feels will better help me deal with issues around self-esteem, especially on the foggy days.

30th October – Canterbury

My annual 25-minute check-up at the GP's surgery with nurse Angela for my blood pressure and a chat. Whilst my relationship with my GP is positive, I feel at times like this that I would prefer that he conducted this check-up, as there are questions I would like to ask but am unable to do so.

3rd–5th November – Telford

Following previous attendance at United Kingdom Dementia Congresses at Brighton, today Rosemary and I ventured north to the Midlands supported by Alex, Lewis and Reinhard.

During the course of Congress, as well as attending a series of, as always, excellent talks and being able to network with so many professional and personal friends, I delivered a workshop with former students and now assistant psychologists Lewis and Alex. We explored how the envoy role has developed alongside the Forget Me Nots before moving on to a critical examination of the key factors and resources required to effectively involve people with dementia and what might motivate them to get involved, and then concluding by outlining the positive and negative impacts of involvement upon the service user. I was also honoured to help launch Congress by speaking from the main stage in the debate on how dementia care has improved (or not) in the past ten years.

12th November – London

After a little break it was back to service user training at Devon House, again led by Lisa and myself, and this time I was supported by Kate Taylor, who is Canterbury's Alzheimer's Society dementia support worker. I didn't know Kate and her role existed until a matter of days ago when I was struggling to find support for this event, and it was suggested I contact the Alzheimer's Society because no student was available. From this, Kate emerged, and we've had a really good day together with her fully engaged in the training and talking on the train.

18th November – Canterbury

Continuing my engagement with the IDEAL project, today Rosemary and I were visited by Dr Alex Hillman and her colleague, Hannah, from Cardiff University. Alex's job is to help lead the research team in gathering the qualitative data from the large cohort of participants in the IDEAL project. She wanted to talk to Rosemary and me, both together and separately, in trying out questions for the questionnaire before taking it out to members of the whole project.

19th November – London

We always use a taxi to travel the two miles from home to Canterbury West station, and I do get terribly anxious some days as the arranged time for it to pick me up approaches. Will it be late? Have they forgotten me? Often they will send a text when it is on its way, but not always. The call centre for the local company we use is based in Albania and the girls there have now got to know me and most are very understanding as I do explain the difficulties that dementia presents. Some days I have walked around outside our house anxious and foolishly thinking this might speed the taxi up.

Linked to feelings of uncertainty and anxiety, I do feel that my days are numbered as a member of the Royal College of Psychiatrists executive committee and that by us establishing a patient forum of three patients with various mental health conditions I can ease out quietly.

20th November – London and Canterbury

Reinhard, Chris and I, supported by Lewis and Vishy, one of this year's students, have been invited by the organisers at University College to give a service user perspective on young onset dementia. This, I'm told, was a departure for the organisers, because previously conferences had always been totally orientated around professional speakers, and most of the audience – if not all – have been professionals in the past. We felt we were breaking new ground by agreeing to speak.

A new departure for the Forget Me Nots, which was to utilise the interest and skills of Martin, one of our members, as a historian in taking us around our city to visit some of the key sites – primarily the cathedral and its precincts. There were six Forget Me Nots on the walk, plus three supporters. It was a really interesting day and we were grateful to Martin for leading.

26th November – London

Maybe the therapy is helping because I have been experiencing fewer foggy days lately. A very full day. Rosemary and I attended the annual VALID (Valuing Active Life in Dementia) occupational therapy project advisory group meeting in the morning. We then walked from the venue in Euston to St Pancras where we met Reinhard. Rosemary travelled home to Canterbury on her own whilst Reinhard and I went on to the Alzheimer's Society for our quarterly DAA meeting. Possibly too much in the one day, but I did feel well and enjoyed the stimulation of the meetings.

27th November – Middlesex

After yesterday, an early start with the support of Briony, one of this year's placement students, travelling to the West Middlesex Hospital, to participate in the monitoring of the PREVENT research project. This is the third time I've done this, and I really am keen to be involved in this role because this project is important, as it continues to examine how people can possibly better prevent the onset of dementia in their 50s, 60s and early 70s.

After this meeting Briony boldly supported me in dashing across London to attend a creative arts in dementia event being organised by Southwark DAA. They had asked me to talk to attendees about writing and I was delighted that Liz Jennings joined me for this. I also sat in on a discussion about the importance of music for people with dementia chaired by Veronica from Arts 4 Dementia. I mentioned to the group that I hadn't played my guitar since being diagnosed as I felt sure I would now be rubbish compared to before the onset of dementia. Saddened by this, Veronica and others tried to encourage me; one suggestion she made was that I should take on the challenge of learning a new instrument so that then I would not be influenced by my past skill level.

30th November – Canterbury

Having spoken to the students a couple of months ago as a group and having been up to London now with Briony, Vishy and Nicki, today was the first opportunity to meet at my house with Michael and Kai, the two students who will be providing me with one session a month of support with writing and using the computer at my home. Later this afternoon, I met with Nicky Thompson from Canterbury City Council, who was keen to talk with me about a creative writing project that she plans to run in Canterbury. She is looking for support in recruiting people with dementia, and also hoped that maybe I might be able to attend as a participant. I told her that if my diary allows it, I will. I have the dates, and hopefully I'll be able to get along to some.

3rd December – Canterbury

Starting to explore compassion-focused therapy (CFT) with Dr Yvette Kusel. I am confident with Yvette that this will help me and provide the springboard to recovering my health back to where it was 18 months ago. She gave me a helpful handout with the CFT model illustrated. It has three key elements: a person's 'threat system', 'drive system' and 'care-giving system'.

She assures me that this is not a 'quick fix' and that I will require ten sessions and then a review. I am up for this and see it fitting closely alongside the 'Kitwood flower' which I carry with me everywhere in my diary. I said to Yvette that I don't have any tattoos but if I did then the Kitwood flower would be the one I would go for!

4th December – Canterbury

As part of the Forget Me Nots group, I've been invited to be filmed by KMPT for their website as part of a project called Live It Well Library. The idea is to film service users who are living with a range of disabilities and mental health issues, then placing that film on the Mental Health Trust's website so that interested people can access it.

It went really well, and watching it back this evening, the part of the interview that has stayed with me is towards the end, when I am asked to give advice to other people with dementia about living well: what would be my key thoughts and advice around that? Part of it was around living in and for the day, but also having something achievable in the near future to look forward to.

8th December – London

The full network meeting of the Young Dementia Network steering group with Rosemary and Reinhard, after which we stayed overnight in a hotel because we have an early start tomorrow in London again for the DAA's annual meeting, which is being held at the Russell Hotel.

9th December – London

After a pleasant evening meal with Rosemary at the Russell Hotel, which is decorated profusely ready for Christmas, I was able to engage and participate comfortably in the DAA's annual meeting today.

After the recent sad loss of Richard Taylor, even closer to home and just as sad and significant a loss is the recent passing of Peter Ashley. Peter was a giant of a man in so many ways and was for many years the sole voice of those of us with a dementia. I was humbled and honoured to share the stage today in delivering a tribute to Peter alongside Professor Dawn Brooker.

Here is the tribute I wrote and delivered today:

'Peter always referred to people with dementia and their carers as being the two sides of the same coin. I'm afraid that my wife and I need to leave the conference after this tribute in order that she can attend an event which is important to her this evening, and I am meeting a friend. Enjoying life outside of dementia is as Peter would agree also very important for us both. I am honoured and pleased, though rather humbled, to have been asked to contribute to this tribute today to our dear friend Peter. I would like my piece to be seen as a thank you to him.

Firstly, I have known Peter really well for four years and I wish to express my thanks for his humour, intellect and wisdom which always is a powerful combination, especially when found in a friend and ally.

Secondly, to say thanks to him for asking the questions many of us thought about but lacked the confidence to ask, and for those questions which never occurred to us because we didn't have the benefits of his insight or experience.

Thirdly, thank you Peter for holding the professionals to the tasks they needed to address by teaching them what it really is like to live with a dementia. 'A', though a short word, was a big word when used by Peter, and he was A big man. A pioneer, an advocate in the truest sense of the word and the first to pick up the baton [hold up relay baton acquired from local primary school!], move forward with it and, as a part of his legacy, pass it on. Many aspire to leave the world a better place than when we arrived, although few achieve this. Thank you sincerely Peter for giving hope to us all who follow on from you that through your efforts and success, maybe we can also achieve this. I am proud that along with George, Lorraine, Tommy, Trevor and Peter we are here today to pick it up and to build upon his lasting contribution.

Once again, thank you Peter. Thank you everyone.'

12th December – Rochester

Following last year's initial Alzheimer's Society Carols by Candlelight service in London, they are now taking this around the country to a number of cities. I was asked by Jane Cotton from the society if I would prepare and deliver a talk at Rochester, which I have been happy to do. I entitled the talk 'The Lion, the Sun and the Christmas Card', which was inspired by C.S. Lewis and the meetings I have with Eric and Jen.

16th December – Maidstone

A KMPT Young Onset Dementia Network meeting led by Reinhard during which we discussed in detail our Trust's provision for younger people with dementia.

17th December – Canterbury

Today's therapy appointment with Yvette was very constructive and has hopefully set me up for a good Christmas. More sessions are planned for 2016 where we can work together using CFT. This set me in a reflective mood tonight. I am scribbling down my thoughts around 4 Cs – connection, commitment, compassion and consideration equals HOPE – against the 4 Rs – reproach, regret, recrimination and rejection equals HURT. I think this sits alongside the time with Yvette and my ever-present thoughts on the Kitwood flower against malignant social psychology.

23rd December – Canterbury

I have had a lovely 60th birthday today celebrating with my family who I dearly love. The ten of us went to the Parrot pub for a special meal. Sitting in the Parrot opposite our three grandchildren, I am thinking to myself that no granddad could be more proud of their grandchildren than I am of Byron, Rhian and William. Rosemary and I are truly blessed.

Amongst my gifts were a solar watch from Rosemary (the last watch I had was from Gareth for my 40th birthday), and a collection of classic books (she used the word 'classic' to describe the books and me!) from Karon, all of which were first published in 1955, the year I was born.

Lots to read in the new year, and as my diary tells me there are still many interesting projects ahead.

Sometime in 2015

Dear Alzheimer's

I am not being defined by you. I never thought that I'd ever quote W.C. Fields, but a statement of his from the 1930s caught my eye recently and seems very fitting to open this year's letter to you. The quote read: 'It ain't what they call you, it's what you answer to that counts.' I am including this in my talks now, and for me this connects to my continued resistance to being defined by you. This links closely to the story I also tell from a conversation with Lewis, a nine-year-old who is one of the children I enjoy hearing read at the local primary school. It is startling how children see people differently from adults, and this helps me to see the future against you more positively. Having seen an article about me in a local magazine, Lewis didn't define me by my dementia; he defined me by seeing my first name.

I take strength from this alongside at last having a care plan which is fit for purpose. It is written by my consultant and me and will be monitored by both of us. It places six key words as headings to help defeat you – 'what' (what I will receive to help me), 'when' (when I will receive it), 'where' (where I will receive it), 'who' (who will deliver it), 'how' (how it will help me against you) and 'why' (the impact of the intervention). I rely upon structure against you, and this for me gives one I can rely upon. It is not rocket science that this will make for a good plan, and I, with help, will do everything I can to maximise the benefits of this plan for as long as I possibly can.

Beyond my care plan I now have a sense of what Bob Dylan meant when he wrote and sang about having God on his side. For too long I have been detached from God and now through Eric and Jen I have gained such positive and sincere insight into faith and life generally that I feel a bit stronger once again. It has helped me deal better with the flaws that you highlight and encourage, and whilst I cannot dismiss them I am better able to address, and learn from, them. I do make mistakes – lots of them – and I sense you are watching and waiting to exploit this. I know, unlike people supporting me, God will always stay with me, and unlike some, God is not at all negative or judgemental. Alongside my allies already known to you I now have a more powerful one for which I feel blessed.

Re-reading my diary I sense that you are trying extra hard after 2014 – the rollercoaster year – to get the better of me. You are not succeeding. You will not take away my spirit or soul, though there are days when you do affect my thinking.

I remember a story from my days as a head teacher which I shared at the Forget Me Nots meeting in September when last year's students handed over to this year's.

One evening, a Native American elder told his grandson about a battle that goes on inside people. He said, 'My son, the battle is between two wolves inside us all. One is anger, envy, jealousy, sorrow, regret, greed, arrogance, self-pity, guilt, resentment, inferiority, lies, false pride and superiority. The other is joy, peace, love, hope, serenity, humility, kindness, benevolence, empathy, generosity, truth and compassion.' The grandson thought for a moment and then asked his grandfather, 'Which wolf wins?' The elder simply replied, 'The one that you feed.'

Wisdom such as this, if adhered to, WILL beat you, 'dear Alzheimer's'.

Your unfaithful host

Keith

2016

—

'Walking and talking with family and friends'

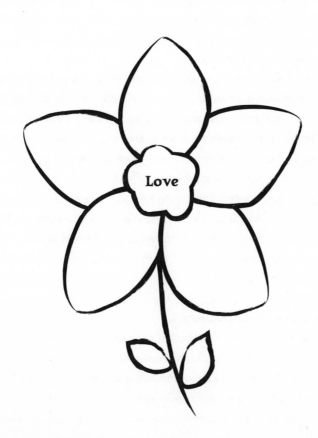

5th January – Canterbury

It's exciting to begin the new year with the final planning meeting for the film project today with Liz Jennings, Rosemary, myself and Frances James, who coordinates University of Kent psychology students on placement and as volunteers. Now the venue is sorted, the films are being chosen by the Forget Me Nots. Liz has prepared a stimulating plan for the discussions of each film, and publicity by poster and word of mouth has generated a lot of interest from people with dementia and supporters. I can almost smell the popcorn after months of planning!

Thinking of the new year, I am delighted to have a new journal from Karon, which has a map of the London Underground on the front cover, so very thoughtful of her. In moving over to the new edition I spent time today reading through previous diaries and journals. Entries are like me – sometimes lucid and sometimes more vague – which I guess is indicative of how I was on the day. Sometimes I wonder – was that really me who did that or said that on that day?

7th January – Canterbury

At my therapy session today with Yvette, our focus was to look at the events I engaged with over Christmas, such as my 60th birthday. We talked about my desire to wear multi-coloured (particularly green) clothing rather than drab dull colours – certainly not a mission to achieve sartorial elegance but a desire to help restore my sense of positive self-image. We considered the importance of small things and how at times they make a big difference to me, both positive and negative.

After this session with Yvette I still felt well enough to attend an envoy review meeting at St Martin's Hospital with Reinhard where we discussed the role during 2015 and we looked forward to its continuation during 2016.

11th January – Canterbury

Liz organised an evening get-together at a local pub for the volunteers who are going to be involved in the cinema project. This gave Rosemary and me an opportunity to meet the others, who are friends of Liz, and to move forward our plans for the now rapidly approaching project.

14th January – London

In order to provide me with effective support I managed to negotiate Lewis's release with Reinhard, his line manager, to support my attendance at the 2020 Expert Reference Group (ERG) which is seeking to establish a post-diagnosis pathway for people with dementia in England. The meeting was again at the Royal College of Psychiatrists. For me this is very important as Lewis has the experience and understanding around the context of this work alongside the potential impact it could have on dementia care in this country. I have a significant sense of responsibility around my role on this project, and being able to share this with Lewis, whom I trust implicitly, settles some of my anxiety.

19th January – Canterbury

After confirming our wish to attend a volunteering and careers evening at the University of Kent, Lewis, Liz and I attended the event at the Psychology School in Keynes College, University of Kent, this evening. Upon arrival, we met Frances James who coordinated the event, and we manned a stall which focused on volunteering with the film project. We got some interest through this, but I felt there was a greater potential if I actually stood up and spoke with the students present. I managed to encourage Frances to give me five minutes to inspire the students to join our project as volunteers. After the talk there was a queue of them wishing to sign up!

20th–21st January – London

Through Claire Thorpe from the Alzheimer's Society, Rosemary and I had been given tickets for a pantomime at Sadler's Wells in London which we attended this evening. It was a charity event for a range of charities and we were there to represent the Alzheimer's Society. The performers came from PricewaterhouseCoopers. They were incredibly talented and it was a really entertaining evening. After the pantomime, we stayed in London for the night, supported by the Alzheimer's Society.

22nd January – Canterbury

After what seems like an eternity of planning, today saw the launch of the film project, beginning the programme with *The King's Speech*. This film went down really well with everyone present. There were about 25 people in attendance, all of whom have a diagnosis or are their carers. Led by Liz, we focused upon the story and the acting in the discussion afterwards, and everybody made constructive comments expressing their individual points of view. People sat wherever they wanted to sit, and of course chose to go with their husbands, wives or whoever was supporting them today. For the discussion element I may well choose to mix up the groups in future as some people spoke on behalf of their 'other half'.

27th January – London

Lisa and I delivered one of our Alzheimer's Society service user involvement training workshops today, and I was supported in travelling up to London and at the event by Chris Norris and Nicki (Nicki being one of the students on placement this year). It was a good opportunity to introduce Chris to the training package that Lisa and I have developed over the last few years. He also participated – both in helping facilitate groups and as a member of a group.

Whenever I visit the Alzheimer's Society in London I feel genuinely welcome and very much a part of the team. I really value and treasure this feeling and hope that it can be sustained even though some of the faces I meet change as some move on to pastures new and fresh professional and personal challenges.

29th January – Canterbury

As I have been very much up and down recently with my mental health, I took my exercise book full of notes to see Yvette today. The foggy days are now much patchier and sometimes more dense – a bit like driving along a road when you travel in and out of clear road and patches of fog. I talked through the notes with her around still finding the atmosphere and interactions at the Forget Me Nots difficult, but to counterbalance that I outlined the benefits that I and others are deriving from the film project. Talking with Yvette certainly helped to restore the 'sun'. Her patience and understanding allow me to explain how I feel and how I attempt to deal with sometimes challenging interactions with others.

Key areas where Yvette is focusing on are my self-esteem and the impact of the Alzheimer's and depression, and trying to manage both of those better than perhaps I have been doing recently. We also spent time discussing how frustrated I feel at times because of dementia as I partly recognise the challenges that it presents to me. Sometimes this is manifested in me talking too much or jumping in when previously I would have been far more patient. She suggested an app called 'Stop, Breathe & Think', which we expect could help me in the future, and then patiently helped me to install it on my phone. It utilises mindfulness, which I am becoming more open-minded about.

3rd–4th February – London

After several weeks of planning and communication between Age UK and myself, Rosemary and I attended an international symposium on ageing at Age UK's headquarters. It was a really stimulating event, which brought together bankers and social care alongside those from the legal fraternity in discussing ageing well and how older people can be supported to maintain their independence. I have been asked to speak at the event around living well with dementia, and I took with me the *Welcome to Our World* book, which I was able to promote and sell. It was interesting to work with Age UK in London for the first time. I was most impressed by their staff who supported me in this venture, namely Lea Renoux.

5th February – Canterbury

The first film in the movie project, *The King's Speech*, went down extremely well. Today's was again chosen by the Forget Me Nots and was *The Monuments Men*. Not such a good film, and chosen by a number of men at the Forget Me Nots who didn't actually attend, hence the flaws of democracy in action. The story is a bit contrived and was very American in its approach. It didn't go down terribly well with the audience, which was a shame.

8th February – London

Rosemary joined me for the final meeting of the Truth Inquiry at the Mental Health Foundation. Today's event was designed to bring together professionals and service users as a conclusion in order to discuss the production of the document that is going to result from the two years we've been working on this investigation. The meeting was led by Professor Graham Stokes, Dr Daphne Wallace and Toby Williamson, and our discussion will hopefully support Toby's efforts towards producing the final report, which I and others await with great interest.

9th February – Whitstable

Whilst Rosemary attended her weekly art lesson in the town, I took myself on my frequent beach walk and used it as an opportunity to call in and see Jocelyne to chat about her doctoral thesis which I am helping a little with. The beach walk is an important part of my weekly routine and I follow the same route each time but will, from time to time, challenge myself a little by doing the route in reverse.

Whitstable is a lovely seaside town with lots of small independent shops. When the tide is in, the harbour is an attractive working harbour and the beach area becomes a really pretty location, whereas when the tide is out it is less attractive and appears very muddy. It has many independent shops and cafés which I applaud, but then rather hypocritically use Costa's each time because I am a creature of habit.

11th February – Canterbury

The feeling of being up and down with my health continues. Today I saw Yvette, for what was the seventh therapy session with her. We discussed how taking medication helps me live well with dementia, and how for the first time recently I've thought about not taking it because then maybe it would be easier to blank out the problems that I face. We also discussed how I find shopping difficult (such as buying shirts), with the choice being overwhelming in shops such as Marks and Spencer. We moved on to talk about how I strive to put things right and keep everybody happy and in harmony. I seek forgiveness for any upset I may cause inadvertently, through error or being stupid, saying or doing the wrong thing. As always, we went back over the previous session and Yvette picked out the various points that she wanted to re-emphasise with me, focusing on the positive but seeking to address 'here's where I'm worried and concerned'.

16th–18th February – Windsor

As it's school half-term holiday, Rosemary and I went to look after William, our grandson. Nick, his father, was at work and Karon was on a week's holiday in her favourite place, Hong Kong, a Christmas present from Nick.

We went over to Windsor to spend time with William, which we as always really enjoyed.

22nd February – London

Tricia Fincher, the Kent community librarian working with older people, and myself attended the launch of a project by the charity The Reading Agency called Reading Well, held at the Big Lottery headquarters. This project is being funded by the lottery over a number of years, seeking to use books as a means of tackling loneliness in older people through establishing a large network of reading friends. It builds upon Books on Prescription which I have been involved with over the past two years. Whilst dementia isn't the main focus of the project (it is really focusing on loneliness and isolation in the elderly), clearly there will be overlaps, and I've been invited along to bring the lived experience of dementia to this piece of work.

25th February – Canterbury

For some time KMPT and the Forget Me Nots have been concerned about being able to provide support for members of the group during the summer period when students are no longer available. In the past we've been fortunate to have some short-term financial help for this from DEEP. Now we're at the stage where we want to formulate a bid to DEEP to secure funding for a member of staff who will coordinate support for the Forget Me Nots, and any other groups that come into existence in the area, alongside providing additional support to that which is available from students. I shared my experience and opinions at the meeting today with the professionals, supported by Kai (one of the placement students). The points made at the meeting will be taken away and a bid formulated, which will be shared with us before presenting to DEEP.

26th February – Canterbury

A very busy day. It began with an appointment at the hospital for therapy with Yvette and was then followed by meetings at Café Solo and Thanington Resources Centre with Liz and Rosemary, after which Rosemary and I watched a performance of *Joseph and the Amazing Technicolour Dreamcoat* at the Marlowe Theatre in the afternoon. Gee, what a busy day. I felt well though. Consequently I was able to engage in each of those four activities.

No trip to Australia this year for the first time in many years, in fact since 2003 when we went to Vietnam and Thailand instead. Will we go back to our beloved Australia again? I'm not sure. Rosemary and I have talked about this at some length and it's something I spoke to Yvette about today. The reason I'm not sure about going is that the trip last year was, generally speaking, very good but there were challenges that had previously not been so noticeable. I also wish to ensure that memories of this important part of our life remain positive and are not brought into question from negative experiences being had. Rosemary's reason for not being sure about going again is largely around the distance and the time it takes to get there and back and the subsequent impact that jet lag has upon her.

28th February – Canterbury

After a number of encouraging conversations with Eric about attending a service at Barton Church, today I was able to do so, and was invited to give a short talk on the theme of 'This time tomorrow' as part of a sequence of talks at the church. There were approximately 150 people in the congregation and I enjoyed the camaraderie of the event, the service, the music (which was very modern) and the feeling of optimism, energy and positivity within the room. It was a very different audience to speak to. The majority there were younger people but with a significant smattering of oldies as well. Afterwards, when having coffee, Jean, a former colleague of mine from the 1980s, came over and we had a lovely catch-up.

29th February – London

Having now become more settled in my role within the Dementia Action Alliance board, sharing the role of 'Person with Dementia' with Tommy Dunne, today's meeting was very straightforward. I was able to engage in the discussion and the topics that we discussed. I had Reinhard's engaging support on the journey and during the meeting, then afterwards was able to spend a little time with Lisa and Katie from the Alzheimer's Society – a real treat to be able to catch up with them.

1st March – Canterbury

As part of my role within the IDEAL project, I had agreed that one of the senior researchers, Dr Alex Hillman from Cardiff University, could come and visit us to discuss the project and the questions that the 1500 participants would be asked. Alex's role was to use me alongside a small number of other people as a sounding board before completing the final version of the questionnaire, which will inform the research project. Alex was delightful and very conscious of working with people affected by dementia. She spoke to Rosemary and me together to start with, and then at greater length to us separately. It's a real privilege to be able to influence in such a way this important piece of work.

2nd March – London

Another constructive Young Onset Dementia full network meeting with Rosemary and Reinhard where I feel very valued, respected and involved. It is so important to raise the profile of those of us with young onset – for far too long 'youngsters' like myself with dementia have had such a rough deal from services.

3rd March – London

In my role as part of the Alzheimer's Society Research Network panel (focusing upon care and wellbeing), I attended one of the twice-yearly meetings in London today with the support of Kai, one of the students. It's worth noting that the budget available to be allocated for research projects from the Alzheimer's Society through the network has increased from £2 million per year when I joined in 2012 to £8 million this year, with an expectation of £10 million in 2017. Thankfully the quality and quantity of care projects have improved markedly since the network was split into bio-chemical and care, so between 30 and 40 per cent of the budget can now be allocated to care with a possible ambition of rising to close to 50/50, which would be amazing.

4th March – Canterbury

The third film in the movie project chosen by members of the Forget Me Nots is *Paddington*. Both Liz and I were pleasantly surprised how well it went down. I think part of that was down to the discussion we had afterwards, where the focus areas ranged from family issues exposed within the film through to looking at the plight of refugees and equating the character of Paddington to that of refugees, who are very much in the news today.

8th March – Manchester

As part of the ERG project with Lewis, he and I attended a meeting today at Manchester University. It was an incredibly early start and a late arrival home afterwards. I'm not sure what I was able to contribute. All I can remember, although it was barely a few hours ago, is a conversation that Lewis had in the taxi with a lady and a gentleman where the guy had dementia and the lady was his wife. Lewis was asking them about the day, and neither of us was convinced that the guy had contributed or gained anything from the day as he had remained silent throughout. His wife had been quite vocal, but it was he who was listed as a member of the group, and not her. This in my mind creates an extra pressure on me because two people with dementia in the context of this meeting became one.

11th March – Canterbury

Today Reinhard and Elizabeth had arranged for 16 Forget Me Nots members with support to have an extended meeting, brought about by a request from Essex University for feedback on a piece of work that they wish to take to the United Nations.

Prior to the meeting I was asked to meet and greet Anne Marie, a new member of the group who I think will be an interesting addition to the Forget Me Nots, someone who I'm sure will participate fully in the months and years ahead.

14th March – London

Following on from the Research Network panel meeting 11 days ago, today I attended the board meeting at the Alzheimer's Society headquarters. Each board meeting has four members from the lay panel representing the views of the panel and of the Research Network generally. We sit alongside approximately ten academics from universities around the country and we discuss the projects that are potentially fundable or which we deem fundable. One project that stood out for me today was The Angela Project, which is seeking to improve the situation regarding diagnosis and post-diagnostic support in the area of young onset dementia, something I feel passionately about and advocate for. I was asked to speak on behalf of the project and I did so enthusiastically and, I hope, eloquently. This seemed to engage with the board and helped achieve their support for the project which I hope will be funded.

18th March – Canterbury

The next film project showing was *Mao's Last Dancer*. This was thought to be a very challenging film for the group because it is one that no one will have ever heard of since it comes from Australia and hasn't been released over here in the UK, either through the cinema, DVD or TV. I did though see the wonderful book in Waterstones recently. Approximately a third of the dialogue is in Chinese, and two-thirds in English. The film has a cast that no one present would relate to as they wouldn't know any of the actors. The film also uses flashback, which one would anticipate people with dementia would find challenging and I'm sure that we do. Because of the beauty of the cinematography, the strength of the story and the characterisation of the main players, the film was incredibly well received by the group. Rosemary was especially pleased as it is one of her favourite films. I think that Liz's discussion topics based upon the strengths of the film really helped with this.

20th March – London

A rare tourist trip up the capital to the Royal Academy where there is currently a Monet exhibition. Rosemary and I thought this was a lovely way of celebrating our 35th wedding anniversary tomorrow.

22nd March – London

Another very relaxing 'jolly', this time up to Elstree Studios with the Canterbury Arts Society through our friends John and Jean to see a filming of the TV show *Pointless*.

23rd March – London

DAA quarterly meeting at the Royal College of Occupational Therapy attended with Canterbury's Alzheimer's Society dementia support worker Kate Comfort (née Taylor). An eclectic, interesting mix of presentations on issues such as the LGBT (lesbian, gay, bisexual, transgender) community, intimacy and dementia, and closing with a session on the cultural perceptions of dementia. As always at these events I learn such a lot, not just about dementia but about broader societal issues.

1st April – Canterbury

The final film in the project at Thanington Resource Centre was *A Walk in the Woods*, based upon a book written by Bill Bryson, with Robert Redford playing the part of Bill. The film was well received by the 28 people present and was a good closure to the project. I have been thrilled to witness Liz's growth in confidence during this project and to watch the absolutely positive responses of all who have attended the sessions. There were no fools around today on 1st April! Such a breath of fresh air and immensely motivating to do more projects with Liz and people affected by dementia.

That was this morning, then after lunch at home, Rosemary and I went to an exhibition at the Beaney with Sumita Chauhan, a friend of mine, who visited me a little while ago to discuss her PhD on digital sculpture. She has completed the work with a group of elderly people with dementia, all of whom were over the age of 80. What they have produced is staggering and very, very moving: an absolutely fabulous exhibition of digital sculpture created by people who would never have dreamed it was possible.

7th April – London

It's amazing how time seems to fly by, and it is almost frightening that a year ago I was at the same place at the same time; the place being St James's Palace, and the event being the Alzheimer's Society awards. This year I was asked to present flowers as a thank you to the Alzheimer's Society patron, Her Royal Highness Princess Alexandra. When doing so, going through my mind repeatedly was the statement 'Say Ma'am as in jam' to the point where I have to say I was concerned I would have a slip of the tongue and refer to HRH as 'jam'! Another highlight for me was to spend time in conversation with Richard Madeley who was MC for the day.

11th April – Canterbury

Liz Jennings, Nada and I, supported by Kai and Michael (the two placement students working closest with me this year), met to prepare and begin to write an application for the UK Dementia Congress. We are seeking to take the movie project to Congress this year because we feel it is such an innovative and interesting piece of work and that it could engage with a wider audience.

12th–13th April – Bristol

I've never been to Bristol before, so I was excited by the prospect of travelling over there with Rosemary. We were invited to attend a workshop being organised by the RSAS (Royal Surgical Aid Society) who had hired the

Penny Brohn Centre for a workshop and had facilitated Rosemary and me staying there. The Penny Brohn Centre is one set up to support people living with cancer and the RSAS are looking to create a similar centre somewhere else in the UK, which will focus on the needs of carers of people with dementia. The centre is set up on holistic grounds, with food and drink that best supports this, plus the rarity of no television or internet in their bedrooms. Also, whilst we were in Bristol, Rosemary and I used the opportunity to have lunch at a local pub with Becca, one of our nieces, who lives and works in Bristol.

19th April – Canterbury

Because I'd been feeling very tired lately and was finding difficulty getting support for a visit into London to attend the DAA board meeting, I opted to phone in. I found the experience extremely challenging because, when I've done a phone-in in the past, I have been in a small group and have been encouraged at times to speak. On this occasion it was a much larger group, and alongside how I feel with my dementia at times, being able to contribute was much harder. Consequently, I don't think I would wish to do this again.

20th April – London

With Lewis's support I attended another ERG meeting in London today as part of that ongoing piece of work. One area of focus to which I was able to contribute with Alistair Burns's encouragement was around care plans. My plan has as its headings *What*, *When*, *Where*, *Who*, *Why* and *How* and is structured around these key words to enable me to live as well as possible. I explained that my care plan took four years to get and ten minutes for my consultant and me to write. In my view all those diagnosed should have a fit-for-purpose plan as soon as is appropriate after their diagnosis and certainly within six months.

21st April – London

Through Matt Murray at the Alzheimer's Society, I was invited today to give what was termed an 'inspiring talk' to the operations team in the Alzheimer's Society. I thought that, rather than doing a straightforward talk, what might be more interesting and a little different would be if

Matt and I did a conversation, whereby it would be structured around an interview. Matt would prompt me with questions focusing not only on my involvement with the society but also beyond this, and it gave me a platform to promote Welcome to Our World, which I am feeling is drawing to a close for me. Over the last couple of weeks, Matt and I prepared this together through email and telephone. It went really well, and both of us enjoyed it. Afterwards, Rosemary, Matt and I went for a pleasant lunch.

22nd April – Canterbury

As the movie project is drawing to a close, it is clear that everybody wants something more, and people are sad that it's coming to an end. The other day I called into the local Odeon cinema in Canterbury to pick up some copies of their silver screen programme which I could then take to encourage Forget Me Nots in their current desire to see modern films. Sitting there waiting for some to be printed, I noticed a poster advertising the movie *Eddie the Eagle*, which is soon to come to Canterbury. I asked if the manager was available, to which I was told he was. He came out and we had a conversation about the project, which he had heard of through Liz. He supported my view that it would be good to have an additional bonus seventh session at the cinema when we could watch the film *Eddie the Eagle*. We could then give the Odeon some feedback on making their showings more dementia friendly. We did this today. I secured a £100 grant from the Alzheimer's Society to cover the cost and we had total exclusive use of the cinema for the morning's special showing. Everyone really enjoyed the film and we concluded it with one of our discussions, led by Liz and similar to those at Thanington (but without the PowerPoint). Again we discussed what issues the film had evoked for us – largely about being the underdog and living your dream – alongside what we had enjoyed about the film. Liz and I will now write up the project and – if we're successful – take it to Congress at Brighton in November.

26th April – London

At the Alzheimer's Society supported by Briony, one of the students co-delivering the service user training package which Lisa, Claire Garley and I have developed. I love these days as working with Lisa is always a relaxed treat, and the staff accessing the training come with such enthusiasm and commitment to deliver services which better meet the needs of people with dementia.

28th April – London

DEEP have been thinking for some time about bringing together a number of us who are very active nationally in discussing issues that are not always fully covered in DEEP groups. Consequently, they've formed a special group called the DEEP Think Tank, and today was one of those meetings at the Mental Health Foundation, chaired by Steve Milton and Philly Hare. Rosemary and I followed this up with lunch nearby with Gareth our son.

3rd May – Canterbury

Tenth therapy session with Yvette. Halfway through the package of treatment and feeling some of the benefits in my improved wellbeing, especially around relaxation and resilience, which is helping me feel a little more positive about myself.

4th May – Canterbury

Had a lovely meeting today in Canterbury with Adrian Bradley, who is the Alzheimer's Society young onset dementia lead. Adrian's post is funded by money raised from an ITV appeal which took place just before Christmas, called 'Text Santa', and Adrian is doing a great job in moving the society forward in its support and provision for people with young onset dementia. Consequently, because the money came from 'texting Santa', my belief in Santa is somewhat restored!

9th May – London

An uninspiring morning meeting at the Division of Clinical Psychology service user involvement forum, focusing across mental health, where I was the only person with dementia and Reinhard was the only professional working with people with dementia. However, after lunch we headed to the Houses of Parliament, where the day took off positively. We were there to celebrate the Division of Clinical Psychology's 50th birthday within the British Psychological Society. Along with a magnificent cake, which we were able to admire and then enjoy, the conversations were around a range of issues which related to mental health. One conversation I had was with an MP who initially upset me because he came out with the view about 'not looking like I had dementia'. I didn't have an argument with him about this, but simply walked away, calmed down, and then returned to where he and Reinhard were talking. By this time, whether Reinhard had spoken to him about this, or whether he had reflected upon his comment, he was more interested in finding out about my experience of dementia in a more open-minded manner.

Then on the return journey, Reinhard was keen that I be invited to their birthday dinner. I declined because I thought this was something for the professionals to enjoy and, also, I was looking forward to getting back to Rosemary at home, so I didn't take up the kind offer. Reinhard said he'd take me back to St Pancras, but I wasn't happy about this because I thought that if he did he'd miss the start of his dinner. I suggested that he take me to the underground and I would be fine from there. Reinhard duly did that and put me on a Circle Line train. Unfortunately, there was a power failure on the journey near Bank station and the packed train was evacuated. I spoke to the guard making announcements and explained that I have Alzheimer's and needed help to get to St Pancras. He politely told me to wait where I was whilst he cleared the crowds and then he would help me. He soon returned and explained that he would lead me to another platform where a train would take me to the next station, and he would phone a colleague to alert him to my needs and this colleague would be waiting for me to disembark from the rear carriage where he had asked me to sit. The second member of staff would help me get to St Pancras. That is exactly what happened and I felt totally safe and supported. Tonight I will write to Lisa, who is the Alzheimer's Society engagement and participation officer for London, who may be able to share this as a positive case study with Transport for London and the society.

15th May – Canterbury

I'm absolutely amazed and staggered that the YouTube film *Keith Oliver's Story* has passed 20,000 views and is now attracting approximately 150 a week.

16th–20th May – Isle of Wight

This is the second trip to the island in a month, this time to Shanklin. Previously, Rosemary and I had been from the 15th to 18th April with the

Shepherdswell Women's Institute group. This later visit is with Canterbury Active Retirement Club, and whilst not members we have friends who are, and they kindly invited us along.

24th May – Canterbury

In a reflective mood today, I'm thinking back over recent sessions with Yvette which took place on 6th April, 3rd May and today. For some time I have realised that there are some committed people who really care and I'm fortunate to have access to – Yvette and Richard Brown being two examples – but the system that we all experience or endure does not always seem to care. My reflective mood continued this evening with Rosemary, at a Blean staff reunion at the Blean Tavern near the school.

27th May – Hounslow

Kai, one of the students, and I went to support Sarah Ghani, a clinical psychologist, and I spoke at a workshop entitled 'Whose Research Is It Anyway?' that she had organised for people within her Trust to focus on potential psychology research developments that she would like to see introduced. One intention of this was to move away from a primarily medical-focused model of care in order to arrive at a better balance which focuses upon the person rather than the disease.

1st June – Canterbury

Having given a bit of thought in recent months to commencing some new writing, today I've decided to take the plunge and begin a new project where I'm starting to write my own story. To do this I've begun to make a plan, which will involve me contacting 72 friends and family, inviting them to contribute to the book. I feel that after Welcome to Our World, which was very much a team project, I would now like to embark on a solo effort but with friends supporting me. I have discussed this with Nada from Innovations in Dementia and Tim from the Alzheimer's Society, both of whom are prepared to back the venture and to support me. It is a big ask, and to be able to surmount the obstacles and hurdles that are going to be in my way I need to recruit allies and friends to be able to navigate through what I'm sure will be at times turbulent waters.

2nd June – London

Toby Williamson asked me to speak today at a meeting connected to a project called VERDe (Values, Equality, Rights and Dementia). The project is focusing on women who have dementia, so consequently the agenda was very much skewed towards that. There were few men in attendance and I was asked to speak from my perspective about the impact the dementia has on me, as a man. The talk that I wrote and then delivered I entitled 'Venus and Mars', which allowed me to explore to an extent how I saw gender issues relating to dementia and to state that whilst there is a dearth of research on women there is even less on men and dementia.

When Rosemary and I got home last night after the meeting we watched our friends Chris and Jayne Roberts on *Panorama*, which we had recorded, and were captivated by their story of living with dementia, which was told over the period of a year with cameras and film crew and discreetly positioned cameras which captured their story.

3rd June – Canterbury

For the past month I've had a diary note to remind me that today is when Paul Simon's new album will be released, the first that he has produced since 2011. I can't remember ever buying an album on its first day of issue but I have today because Paul Simon is still my favourite artist. My connection to his music goes back to purchasing one of my first ever albums in 1971 which was *Bridge Over Troubled Water* at the price of £1.66. I still have that album, continue to love his music and am inspired by his lyrics.

6th June – Canterbury

Running alongside the Forget Me Nots group, Kate Comfort from the Alzheimer's Society has managed to secure backing for a Service User Review Panel (SURP) group within the Canterbury area and today was our initial meeting, attended by six people with dementia supported by Kate. It was a very relaxed, friendly meeting and the idea of this group is that it will focus for about an hour and a half on just one topic. Those who are involved will each have a platform and an opportunity to speak. I sense that this will work really well. Three of us are from the Forget Me Nots and three don't currently belong to a group, and I feel positive about being involved with a different group of people.

8th June – London

Young Onset Dementia full network meeting at the Esme Fairburn Foundation with Rosemary. Opportunities for the network to influence and impact nationally are increasing and today we were delighted that a dear friend, Kate Swaffer, visiting from Australia, was able to join us to sit in on a large part of the meeting.

9th June – West Middlesex Hospital

Following the trip up to West Middlesex Hospital recently with Kai to speak about research, today was the six-monthly PREVENT monitoring meeting at the same venue. The project is moving forward smoothly with a large number of recruits and now Professor Ritchie is beginning to collect data and information on the risks around dementia and possible strategies to help prevent its onset. The venue is never an easy one to get to and it gave Briony, the placement student supporting me today, and me an extended opportunity to converse and get to know each other better.

10th June – London

Six months ago, Nigel Ward approached me at a DAA meeting to ask if I would be willing to speak at this year's Alzheimer's Show at Olympia. Today gave me that opportunity and I delivered a talk I had entitled 'Dementia from the Inside Out' in the main theatre and then later returned to the same stage to sit alongside eminent academics and professionals for a question and answer session with the audience. This was an extremely big gig, and to accompany it, I was very surprised that Nigel had chosen to use my photo on the front of the brochure. I very much enjoyed the presentations but wasn't so keen on the ambience of the venue, although this was somewhat offset by some interesting stalls and, as always, a great opportunity to network.

13th June – Canterbury

Nicky Thompson from Canterbury City Council, who met with me recently to discuss a writing workshop entitled 'Cabinet of Curiosities' for people with dementia, had invited me to join the group but I wasn't able to due to pressures on my diary. However, I was able to get along today and really enjoyed the couple of hours I spent with the group and was able to participate in the exercises that Nicky set. I think the aim of the course is to be able to produce a book at the end which will have Canterbury City Council's backing, and go some way to follow on from Welcome to Our World by being another illustration of what people with dementia can produce through the written form.

14th June – Canterbury
My annual check-up of blood pressure and to see how I am at the GP surgery with the practice nurse.

15th June – Weald of Kent
Both Rosemary and I were disappointed to hear recently that an innovative project organised and coordinated by BUPA around London's planned Garden Bridge was cancelled and the project is likely to be scrapped. This gave us a free day in our diary, so we elected that we would go for a drive into the Weald of Kent to explore numerous picturesque villages that are situated between Ashford and Maidstone. The sun was shining and it was a gorgeous day which we both enjoyed.

21st June – London
Another one of the service user involvement training days which Lisa and I deliver and again thoroughly enjoyable, very stimulating and allowing me to reconnect to the teacher role. Today I was supported by Vishy, one of the students, who, although very quiet, seemed to enjoy the day. The added component today was that, despite delivering these sessions over quite a lengthy period of time, Lisa was assessed by one of the Alzheimer's Society training assessors and the verdict was, unsurprisingly, that she is doing a great job. I am thrilled and delighted to be a small part of this.

23rd June – Canterbury
After a month or so of wrangling, arguing, dogma, prejudices, lies and accusations within the media, today was a big day for this country, where the country went to the vote to decide whether we would stay in the European Union (EU) or whether we will leave.

I think the vote will be close; my vote went for remain, and I hope that remain will edge it and we will stay in, because I feel that this is best for our country despite all the idiosyncrasies and flaws within the EU. Better to be inside an organisation and trying to change it than sitting on the outside moaning and not benefiting from what the organisation can bring. It has not only divided the country, but also split families where I've seen family members holding polarised viewpoints on the decision.

24th June – Canterbury

I like many are in a state of shock reflecting on the vote yesterday for the country to leave the EU by 52 per cent to 48 per cent. Fortunately I have the opportunity to lighten my mood because Dr Noel Collins, an Australian consultant psychiatrist from one of the London Trusts, visited me at home to discuss a new book that he is writing with Mary, an ex-Alzheimer's Society employee. Aided by a glass or two of Aussie red from a bottle brought down by Noel, it encouraged me to write the foreword to his new book, which is likely to be called *The D-Word*. I said I'd certainly consider it but I'd have to have the whole manuscript sent to me, not just sections of it, so that I can write an honest and accurate piece. He agreed totally with my suggestion, so I look forward to collaborating with Noel on this.

27th June – London

After Rosemary and I enjoyed lunch with Nada and Alex Hillman and the ALWAYS group, we headed on to the IDEAL project advisory group meeting at an office located beside Regent's Canal. The group identity is really building, both within the ALWAYS group and the broader IDEAL project advisory group. Whether we are service users or professionals, each individual is very comfortable in expressing their opinion and providing their expertise to the piece of work.

After the meeting Rosemary and I arranged to meet Mycal Miller at a café in St Pancras. We'd not seen him since a brief chat at the Alzheimer's Show, when we'd arranged a lengthier catch-up, which we enjoyed today. I reminded Mycal of the positive impact that his film had made both on me and on people who'd viewed it, and how it had now attracted over 20,000 views.

29th June – Canterbury

Following on from my previous therapy session on 16th June, this was my 13th with Yvette. Thankfully, it wasn't unlucky 13! I feel more resilient and less self-critical and thus better able to deal with what dementia 'throws at me', and this is due to a significant extent to the support provided through Yvette and these constructive therapy sessions.

30th June – Canterbury

After a month of preparation and contacting friends about my new book, today I had the first planning meeting at Augustine House in Canterbury with April Doyle and Liz Jennings, who have kindly agreed to be my closest allies with the book alongside Rosemary. Of the 72 friends I emailed or spoke to inviting them to contribute, all have said yes and many of them have started to send their contributions back to me, which I'm collating. Starting to write the framework and content of the book, I've now got a title as well. I've decided to call it *Walk the Walk, Talk the Talk*, which seems fitting because of the content of the book and because of my personality. Loyalty for me is always crucial, both personally and professionally, and I'll go through anything to support in a non-judgemental way those people I feel loyalty or a connection, commitment, compassion and consideration towards. All of that, I feel, contributes towards the 4 Cs, which equate to hope. The converse side to that is reproach, regret, recrimination and rejection, those 4 Rs, which, when experienced, lead to hurt. I hope to explore those themes within the book, particularly focusing on the positive.

3rd July – Hampton Court

Rosemary and I had a lovely relaxed time at Hampton Court to celebrate her birthday, and then concluded the day with a dinner in a local hotel, where we were joined by Rachel Niblock from DEEP.

4th July – Hampton Court

Alongside the pleasurable day we had yesterday, the other focus behind our visit is an invitation I received through Rachel to speak at the Health and Horticulture conference being held as part of the Hampton Court Flower Show. The focus this year is on disability, and whilst the agenda was set and sent to Rachel for comment, she made the pertinent point that there was no one with dementia as a disability speaking, and she had someone in mind who she felt would fulfil this role, i.e. me. This was agreed to, and it gave me a platform to speak at the end of the conference passionately about my interest in gardening and how both Rosemary and I adapt to the challenges in the garden which dementia presents and use our beautiful, small garden to keep well. To close my talk I told the audience that recently I had been asked, if I was a flower, which it would be. I chose the daffodil as it heralds spring, which brings an end to winter fogs, and also I would have to be grown in the hills as then my sap could be taken after I have died to give galantamine to help others with the same condition as myself. An emotional, truthful and fitting closure which was very well received by the audience.

In the evening I tweaked and then reused the talk to open a special garden that had been commissioned by the Abbeyfield Society as Rosemary and I had been invited to the opening of this garden, which I noticed had been awarded a silver medal. Alongside this we were able to go and explore the garden exhibits and to look at the trade stalls that were there. In the evening we retired tired but happy to a Travelodge in Kingston.

6th July – Canterbury
Every three or four weeks, Eric and Jen and I meet to discuss theology, life in general and things that both I and Jen are doing. In between sessions Eric sets me reading and thinking homework which I try diligently to complete, and has started to teach me to pray using a prayer journal, which I find immensely supportive. Today marks the one-year anniversary of these meetings. I gain so much from our time together and take much of this with me day to day. Eric has taught me so much about faith, Jesus, God and myself and I so look forward to our hour together as being an example of coming away feeling better than I went in – something I wish could occur more frequently and broadly.

7th July – Canterbury
A routine and straightforward envoy review meeting today when I was joined by Reinhard and Chris to briefly talk through the past year, thus giving us more time to focus on our respective roles within the Forget Me Nots.

8th–17th July – St Agnes, Cornwall
Rosemary and I share a love of the Cornish coast and it was lovely to have a week in a comfortable stone cottage in the picturesque, vibrant St Agnes.

Days on the beach and visiting gardens occupied most of our stay alongside a day ambling around shops in historic Truro.

18th July – Canterbury

Moving my book forward, today I emailed Jane Cotton at the Alzheimer's Society to ask her if she could think of a celebrity who may be willing to write the foreword for my new book. With *Welcome to Our World* she recruited Jo Brand to fulfil this for us, which added enormously to the book, both in content and sales for the Alzheimer's Society. I am not sure this time who she will turn to from her network of celebrity supporters of the society.

19th July – London

With Lewis for the final Achieving Better Access to Dementia Care Services Expert Reference Group (ABA ERG) meeting. Today after lengthy discussions we were able to confirm the details for the national Evidence-Based Treatment Pathway, its implementation guide and the workforce planning tool – a substantial piece of challenging work which I am so honoured to have been involved in and lucky to have had Lewis's knowledgeable insight and support enabled by Reinhard.

20th July – Margate

Chris Norris and I attended an event organised by the local clinical commissioning group at the Glow Centre in Thanet and coordinated by Tanya Clover. We encouraged and challenged GPs in our talk about the importance of their role in the diagnosis process and greater signposting towards more post-diagnostic support for people with dementia in our region. An added bonus for me was that there were a few trade stands there and one of them was manned by an ex-pupil who I taught at Swalecliffe Primary School in the early 1990s.

22nd July – Canterbury

As part of my care at the Bodywell Centre in Canterbury I was recommended to see Lisa Smith, a dietician, who has advised me to go on a course of turmeric and lay off gluten and sugar in my diet. Following this I had a GP appointment and, in the evening, finished reading Kate Swaffer's book *What the Hell Happened to My Brain?*

25th July – Canterbury

Following on from my talk at the Royal Horticultural Society at Hampton Court Flower Show, today Sean from the charity Thrive came to my house to film me in our garden speaking about how gardening is important to me and how it can be utilised in care homes, alongside how they can better use their outside space through taking residents into an attractive living environment and then stimulating all the senses of the residents – sight, smell, touch, sound – and by providing staff with a richer work setting. Rosemary and I were pleased to be joined for the day by Nada, who wished to support this piece of work. In preparing for this whilst doing some weeding in our garden, a flash of inspiration struck me. For some time I have struggled with people who I value needing to leave my circle of friends and supporters. Whilst tidying up a flower bed I suddenly thought that these friends are rather like flowers which enter into my life, brighten and enrich it, and then after time fade; some return later but others cannot, and one tries to retain positive memories of their time. I was so pleased to have thought this and I hope this thinking will be a source of strength to me and something I can positively share with Yvette next time I see her.

1st August – London

Rosemary and I attended a summer meeting of the Programme Advisory Board at the Alzheimer's Society with a number of other ambassadors, where we talked through the future of our involvement in the society and how the Dementia Statements, which summarise the aspirations of people affected by dementia, are being rewritten by the society on behalf of the DAA based upon our rights and movement from 'I' to 'we', all of which is a positive way forward.

2nd August – Canterbury

This morning during my regular beach walk at Whitstable I called in to see Jocelyne, who had contacted me to tell me she'd like to give me something. I was surprised, moved and honoured that this turned out to be a full copy of her doctoral thesis on service user involvement, and the 'icing on the cake' is that she had, amazingly, dedicated the work to me. Wow, I did not expect this at all, and it was a lovely thing for her to do. That set me on cloud nine for my three-monthly appointment with Dr Richard Brown that followed this afternoon. Although we feel my dementia has stabilised and the depression is less tidal wave in its impact, Richard still wants me to see him every three months and I know how lucky I am to have this level of care from him. Interesting that now I refer to it as 'my' dementia whereas before it would be 'the' dementia. Maybe taking ownership will help me better take continued shared responsibility for living as well as possible.

3rd August – Canterbury
Therapy session with Yvette set me up positively for a meeting with Lewis to talk about my new book and writing a piece on the new dementia pathway from a service user and supporter perspective for Alistair Burns and the team at the ABA ERG project.

4th August – London
Reinhard and I went to the DAA board meeting today, and then afterwards I had a meeting with Jane Cotton to discuss the new book and to express my thanks that she'd been able to secure a foreword from TV celebrity Richard Madeley.

5th August – Canterbury
Beautiful day and a wonderful occasion which I felt privileged to be a tiny part of, and so pleased to have been invited and to attend the wedding service of Jen and Tom at St Mary Bredin Church in Canterbury. I sat with Eric, Charley and Michael, her fiancé.

17th August – London
Lisa couldn't get a room big enough for 20 delegates at Devon House as the training is always popular and oversubscribed. Fortunately, she'd managed to book a room at the Wesleyan Chapel, Islington. Michael, a former student who is helping cover this summer period before the new group arrive and start their placement, came with me. It was a really good day, but I was saddened when Lisa told me it would be the last one she would be able to deliver as she is leaving the society to join Cancer Research UK (CRUK). She explained that the reason for this was more the pull of working for CRUK rather than the push of the Alzheimer's Society, because cancer

research is another cause very close to her heart. I hope that she and I will keep in touch because we've got on very well as friends over the years and she's written a super introduction to my new book.

21st–24th August – East Kent
I know the weather in August has not been very good, but we've been blessed this week with some warm sunshine which has enabled Rosemary, Karon, William and me to spend some lovely days together enjoying the beaches at Margate and Joss Bay. We took along with us our body board and were able to go swimming in the sea. Having an eight-year-old grandson like William is a real treat, enjoying time spent sandcastle building, ball games on the beach and swimming.

25th August – London
Rosemary and I were called upon today in my ex-head teacher role to support discussions around an Alzheimer's Society project seeking to involve young people in the work of the society. We are looking to engage schools from reception classes to sixth form, alongside further education colleges, plus the scout and guide movement. By doing so we feel the next generation will have a better understanding of dementia and be less fearful of both the disease and those living with it, some of whom may be known to them.

30th August – Canterbury
I'm enjoying writing my book but some of the typing is becoming quite burdensome for both myself and my computer, so today I was lucky that Michael, even though he has ended his student placement, was able to spend half a day with me, helping to type various sections of the book and to help me with my other information technology (IT) challenges.

5th September – Canterbury
I'm delighted that Judy Ayris from Age UK has been able to establish a monthly coffee morning at Thanington Resource Centre in her role as Age UK's dementia lead for the Canterbury area, and I was able to go along today and enjoy a conversation with Judy as well as with the other people who attended: some new faces, plus many familiar ones.

8th September – Middelberg, the Netherlands

I've never been to the Netherlands before, so today was quite an adventure for Rosemary and me as we went on a coach trip through the Channel Tunnel with the WI group from Shepherdswell, the destination being the beautiful, historic old town of Middelberg. We had a lovely meal and a leisurely browse around the town. It was market day, which added to the atmosphere and the ambience of the place. I bought a new shoulder bag and Rosemary was able to buy some material.

13th September – Canterbury

Despite being the hottest September day since 1911, with the temperature peaking at 34 degrees, today's therapy session with Yvette was not adversely affected by the heat. One area that Yvette and I talked about today was that some evenings I get extra anxious, particularly when I get tired, and have developed the strategy of hugging a cushion. Whilst that is comforting, I would prefer to develop more positive strategies, and one area that I wanted to talk to Yvette about is one that Rosemary and I try to pursue, which is to play games in an evening, such as card games or number games. For many years we used to play Scrabble, but now that's too difficult for me because of the spelling issues I now have.

14th September – Canterbury

Ever since the Channel 4 programme *Grayson Perry: Who Are You?*, which included Grayson Perry making a fractured memory jar and focusing upon Christopher Devas and dementia, I have been hooked on Grayson's work. I later saw the vase and alongside this loved seeing his tapestries and urns at the National Portrait Gallery exhibition. I have followed this up by reading books on his life and work. I like his individuality and his quirkiness, alongside admiring his creativity and talent. Today's U3A talk was a fitting celebration of his work.

15th September – London

Following a recent meeting where we were discussing the dementia-friendly communities and young people's initiative within the Alzheimer's Society, today Rosemary and I were invited to help judge this year's young people's awards. It gave me an opportunity to bring to the judging some of my experience and knowledge gained from 33 years in education. I always find it hard to make judgements on nominees, who are all so worthy of awards. By the time the final four in the category are presented, they all deserve the recognition. However, the role demands we find a winner, which we did with a unanimous decision. After what was an intense and focused couple of hours it was lovely to spend time unwinding and chatting with Jane Cotton over a cup of tea in the staff break-out area in the Alzheimer's Society headquarters. Jane was interested to know how the book writing is coming along. I was able to enthusiastically explain how well it is going.

16th September – Canterbury

Following on from our conversations on the train to the PREVENT monitoring, I was able to arrange a meeting for Briony with Pat Chung, head of the occupational therapy course at Canterbury Christ Church University.

Briony was telling me that one result of her placement is that she no longer really wishes to pursue a career in psychology, but would much rather take up the challenge of becoming an OT. I felt that talking to Pat would potentially open up avenues and doors to her that could utilise her psychology degree, and find routes through courses to achieve an OT qualification. Part of the discussion was spent with the three of us, until I felt it was best to leave and let them talk whilst I went and got myself some refreshment, returning later to join them.

19th–21st September – Nottingham

Delivered a speech today at the Admiral Nursing conference in Nottingham. In my talk I was able to utilise the W.C. Fields quote I had found last year which, although nothing to do with dementia, has a useful interpretation. His statement that 'It ain't what they call you, it's what you answer to that counts' has, I thought, a direct relevance to people such as myself. After the conference Rosemary and I were delighted to meet with my cousin Jane and her husband Ian for a meal.

22nd September – London

Rosemary and I, following an invite from the Alzheimer's Society, formed part of an interview panel for the post of director for the exciting venture of a dementia research institute being established in London from 2020 with a budget of £250 million and an aim to find a cure or disease-stopping treatment by 2025. The four international professors interviewed engendered different responses from me, all of which was consistent with others on the panel. I do hope my favoured candidate gets the job as they were the only one to adequately answer my questions on the importance of care research alongside bio-chemical. He also grasped the human perspective behind the question I asked at the end of each of the interviews based upon an article on the institute in the Summer 2016 edition of the Medical Research Institute's newsletter.

23rd September – Canterbury

Working with the students is an important part of my schedule and they provide a central part of my support network, so today as a part of their placement induction I was delighted to meet with the new cohort alongside Chris Norris. The five of them all seem keen and interested and I look forward to working with them on a range of projects this year.

26th–27th September – Birmingham

An inspiring conference – excellent activities and stirring, engaging speakers. I was delighted to have been asked to deliver a speech to officially launch the national Young Onset Network at this event in the colourful, uplifting setting of the city's Botanical Gardens. At the lunch break Rosemary and I were able to take a little while to enjoy some of the floral displays. The only negative for me was during one of the talks which mentioned someone achieving a higher honorary degree, which diverted my thinking to when I had to curtail my M.Ed. studies when first diagnosed. I made an excuse to Rosemary that I wanted the toilet and was very upset, more so in fact in that moment than when I had been told to 'call it a day at the university', as now I realise what I could maybe have achieved with support and understanding at the time.

29th September – London

Joined Matt and Sarah on an interview panel with Rosemary to seek a replacement for Lisa in the role of engagement and participation officer for the Alzheimer's Society in London. The venue on this occasion was the society's Islington office which is shared with Leader of the Opposition

Jeremy Corbyn. Interestingly, we saw Mr Corbyn taking a call in the street outside his office with no security or minders present.

30th September – London

Day 2 of interviews. Today Rosemary was unable to attend, so I travelled up on my own and was met at St Pancras by Matt, who took me along to the Islington office. I'm delighted that the choice of candidate for the job was unanimous and Elizabeth, I'm sure, will ably fill the big hole left by Lisa.

4th–6th October – Manchester

Although I had sped up to Manchester with Lewis recently, this will provide Rosemary and me with the chance to get to know the city rather better, as I have been asked to speak at the Abbeyfield annual conference. Abbeyfield is a splendid small charity whose focus is upon running care homes, and this will give me the opportunity to help them through my presentation and to meet some new caring people through April Dobson, who is their dementia lead, and who I met at Hampton Court.

12th October – London

Rosemary and I travelled to London today to help judge the National Dementia Awards. This is the first time we have done this and we were both feeling uncertain and nervous. My apprehension was well placed as the category we were asked to judge today involved four very different people affected by dementia – two former carers and two people who are very badly affected by dementia, one of whom was unable to speak to us due to it being a very bad day for her.

17th October – Chartham Hatch

Whilst Rosemary attended her U3A quilting class, I was able to have a lovely morning in the woods at Chartham Hatch near Canterbury with three dormice wardens on a U3A dormice monitoring workshop. In the two-hour walk through the woods, checking the strategically placed nest boxes, we found nine dormice. Each of the eight of us present were taught how to check a number of boxes. It took me back to the residential visits I did with Swalecliffe, Barton and Blean schools at Flatford Mill, where the children did activities around live mammal trapping. In that case we caught numerous voles and wood mice, but I had never seen a dormouse before.

18th October – Canterbury

Pat Chung is leading a new OT research project focusing on the empowerment service in East Kent, and Pat was keen to recruit me to the advisory board alongside three OT staff from the area. To enable me to do this I was supported by Sammi, one of the new cohort of students.

20th October – Canterbury

Having finished writing *Walk the Walk, Talk the Talk* and met with and discussed comments from April and Liz, today is the day that I sent off the manuscript to the printers for publication. I am so proud of the book, and Rosemary's artwork which will form the front cover.

Following on from the last therapy appointment with Yvette, today the focus was on a compassionate image of myself to try and encourage me to form a greater positive view of myself in the way that I view other people positively.

Following this I met with Lewis in town and we travelled up on the bus to the University of Kent where we were given a slot to speak to Year 2 psychology students in order to try and encourage them to sign up for a placement at KMPT with older adults. I was able to challenge their limited understanding of what a person with dementia might present like, and Lewis gave them invaluable insight into his experience of the placement and supervision. Our talk was enthusiastically received and now we await seeing how many will sign up.

25th October – London

Rosemary and I both felt privileged today to be able to attend a meeting organised by the Alzheimer's Society and coordinated by Jane Cotton at the Houses of Parliament. This was designed as an awareness-raising event for MPs. As part of it, Shelagh Robinson eloquently delivered a passionate speech about living with dementia.

27th October – London

I have known senior consultant psychiatrist, author and academic James Warner since I served on the Royal College of Psychiatrists Faculty of Old Age executive committee, and found him to be a very supportive chairman. I feel honoured today to be able to co-present with James some dementia training for bankers at Julius Baer International Bank, followed by a dash across London with Rosemary to attend the launch of 'A Million Hands' with the Scout Association and the Alzheimer's Society at 11 Downing Street. This initiative is designed to recruit and energise the scout movement to support through pledges and action good causes such as the Alzheimer's Society.

1st–3rd November – Brighton

For this year's UK Dementia Congress Rosemary, Liz, Nada and I stayed at the Ship Hotel along with all members of the ALWAYS group. This time at Congress I was busy giving talks on IDEAL/ALWAYS, human rights for the DEEP Think Tank, and the Canterbury cinema project. Congress also gave me a great platform to launch *Walk the Walk, Talk the Talk*, which went down very well.

7th November – Canterbury

Spent the day writing and listening sadly to the music of Leonard Cohen who passed away today. He certainly can claim to have helped make the world a better place for many people through his music and poetry, all of which lives on.

8th November – Canterbury

In therapy today with Yvette we talked about people asking how I am. I told her my usual response is either 'I'm doing well' or 'Okay', even if I'm not. I am uneasy about this, so now I often simply thank people for asking on the foggier days because I really want to be honest and truthful with them.

11th November – London

Following our presentation at Congress in Brighton recently, the Think Tank had a stimulating and positively challenging meeting exploring the rights of people affected by dementia with the result that we are seeking, with Philly and Steve's support, to produce a comprehensive document on the subject.

12th November – Canterbury

Today was a fabulous day for me and I was on cloud nine. It was the main book launch of *Walk the Walk, Talk the Talk* at Canterbury Christ Church University, and I was superbly supported throughout the day by April,

Reinhard, Rosemary and Lewis. We were joined by over 70 supporters coming from London or the local area, many of whom had written contributions for the book, and most stayed for an hour or so. During the day I did four timed 20-minute presentations and readings from the book, supported by a photographic backdrop taken from the book and created by April. At the end of each session and in between I signed and sold copies of the book and chatted with dear friends who had kindly come along. To think I needed persuading by April and Liz to do the event as I thought no one would be interested, and that after the success of the Welcome to Our World launch this would be a let-down. I was wrong; the five hours devoted to it today makes up one of the best days of my life, alongside my wedding day, James's birth, Karon and Gareth's wedding and Forest twice winning the European Cup. Certainly the best day for the last ten years!

15th November – London
DAA board meeting with Reinhard, and then met Rosemary at Monsoon at St Pancras before rushing off to an Alzheimer's Society ambassador event with her in the evening at the Gherkin, where I met Bill Turnbull from the BBC, and Rosemary and I stayed the night in London.

16th November – London
After a lovely evening Rosemary and I met with Matt Murray and Chris and Jayne Roberts at the new Alzheimer's Society headquarters to talk about plans for the 3 Nations Dementia Working Group, and to view and then give feedback on the dementia friendliness of the society's new office at Crutched Friars. Plans for the working group are developing well, with the three of us and Hilary Doxford seeking to establish the ground plan and Matt, with our suggestions, looking to recruit another nine people with dementia from around the three nations of England, Northern Ireland and Wales.

17th November – London
An extra ABA ERG meeting in London with Lewis to prepare for the national launch of NHS England and NICE implementation guide *Implementing the Dementia Care Evidence-Based Treatment Pathway*. A lot of hard work by a lot of people which I hope will benefit an awful lot more people!

18th November – London

Rosemary and I joined Becca from the Alzheimer's Society to add the finishing touches to their Young Person Project which is seeking to build upon work within the Dementia Friendly Communities initiative.

21st November – Canterbury

Met Liz at Café Solo with another idea for a project exploring her idea of people with dementia writing an individual film script. It will be a ten-week course called Dreams and Visions. Again another exciting, innovative and original idea and a challenge to focus upon in 2017 with members of the Forget Me Nots in Canterbury and Sunshiners, a similar group of people based in Dover.

In the afternoon I didn't feel well. For some time I have wondered, if I was unwell and Rosemary wasn't available to help, then who would I turn to? I had thought that the police were the obvious source of help. Today Rosemary was having her hair done when I felt wobbly and disorientated in Canterbury. I made my way to the police station. When I arrived there I was confronted by a civilian front-desk clerk who was not at all helpful, telling me that everyone was busy, and when I explained more about my Alzheimer's he got a piece of copier paper and scribbled my name and address. I insisted he had my phone number and then he ushered me out of the station. No offer of a drink of water. No offer to call my wife or get someone to check I was okay. I thought this response – or lack of one – was very poor, and it has undermined my faith and hopes for support from them in future.

22nd November – London

VALID OT project meeting with Polly, a student, then we spent a little time in the British Library, which as a student from Bulgaria she was immensely impressed with, before heading home mid-afternoon.

24th November – London

Another constructive Young Onset Dementia Network meeting, with one focus being upon those of us on the ABA ERG sharing this crucial piece of work with others and seeing how young onset dementia is a part of the way forward for the dementia pathway.

25th November – London

Kristina, who is currently ably supporting me with the PREVENT project, attended with me a special conference for the project at Doggett's, a pub near Blackfriars. A bonus for me was spending some time with an ex-member of Alzheimer's Society staff, Becky Driscoll, and meeting her dad, who is a participant in the project.

29th November – Canterbury

Today's therapy session with Yvette centred upon *Walk the Walk, Talk the Talk*, which we discussed for the full hour. Part of the time focused upon her reflections on reading the book. Her initial trail of thought was around a scenario which involved a break in a friendship and then a reconciliation during my time at university.

30th November – London

A lovely day spent attending the Dementia Friendly Community Awards in London with Rosemary, where I was asked to present the Young Persons Award alongside Angela Rippon. Minister of Health Jeremy Hunt gave the keynote as the event was in Westminster. We'd been invited because of our involvement in the Young Person's Project (the Prime Minister's Champion Group on Dementia Friendly Communities coordinated by the Alzheimer's Society), and the winner was a primary school from Wales.

A sumptuous meal was part of the event and on our table were the nominees for the award I was to announce. I knew the winner and couldn't pronounce it as it was a long Welsh name. I asked the head to tell me her school name, which I wrote down phonetically. Oh gosh, I thought, I've given the game away, so quickly I thought and asked the other nominees to tell me how they would wish their school to be announced if they won! Phew – got away with this as I checked with the winner afterwards and she completely assured me that she didn't twig what I was doing!

1st December – London

The main focus at today's DAA meeting at 1 Whitehall Place was a rights-based approach to dementia care. I was asked to lead a table discussion on seldom-heard groups and rarer dementias.

2nd December – Whitstable

After being involved in the EKIDS group since its inception four and a half years ago, Rosemary and I feel that although we have gained a lot from being a part of the group by way of friendship and sharing information, we've now outgrown it. We've continued our membership for a little while out of loyalty but we feel we need more to continue this commitment into the new year, especially with a very congested diary.

7th December – London

A really stimulating IDEAL project meeting alongside Rosemary, Reinhard and Nada. I totally subscribe to its aims and ambitions around researching what best enables people affected by dementia to live as well as possible, and the constructive interactions that there are between professionals and service users at these meetings. This is public and patient involvement (PPI) at its best.

8th December – Canterbury

Attended an envoy review meeting at St Martin's with Reinhard and Chris. I feel there has been great support from Reinhard to Chris and me, but beyond that now it's questionable what KMPT are able to offer us beyond the placement students – which sadly is very different from how things were in the first two to three years.

9th December – Canterbury

Prior to the Forget Me Nots meeting, I had the Meet and Greet duty. Today the new member was Carol, who I think and hope will be a positive addition to the group. She's got a great willingness to learn and to participate and I'm sure will gain a lot from, and bring a lot to, the group.

12th December – London

A 'foggy day'. Consequently, back home this evening, frustratingly, I have little recall of the MSNAP conference at the Royal College that I attended with Rosemary.

13th December – Canterbury

Myself and a small group of Forget Me Nots supported by Sammi and Celina (placement students) met Pat Chung with Grace Lee and Harrison

Hong from Hong Kong, who are practising OTs over there, to talk to them about our Forget Me Nots group, and the care and support we get for our dementia. The visitors explained how fascinating the Forget Me Nots sounded and how there is nothing similar in Hong Kong. They said they are inspired by us and would take back the idea to their country.

16th December – London

Following the recent project conference I was again supported by Kristina at the six-monthly PREVENT meeting at its West Middlesex Hospital base. After the monitoring meeting I met with Katie Bennett to discuss how the book was selling and to hear how her new job is going at the Alzheimer's Society.

20th December – Canterbury

Alongside talking about my book again, today's therapy session with Yvette looked at setting me up for the Christmas break. Amongst her suggestions which sat alongside my thinking were to try and relax, take a break from the envoy/ambassador role and to enjoy the company of our family. I am looking forward to all of this.

But before taking the break, having arrived home from therapy and taking 30 minutes to grab some lunch – old habits die hard, after 33 years of rushed school dinners and duties – it was straight into a teleconference regarding setting up the 3 Nations Dementia Working Group, which involved myself, Hilary, Chris and Matt Murray from the Alzheimer's Society. The project is making good progress and we are sharing ideas and discussing constructive thoughts about the formation of the group using elements of my planning questions – what, when, how, where and who. I am sure that this will be one of the new, exciting ventures I am looking forward to being involved in during 2017.

Sometime in 2016

Dear Alzheimer's

As I sit at my desk I recognise that you have moved me into a reflective mood. Part of this has seen me looking back over the past five years, and part has focused me on considering my future. I do try to take each day as it comes whilst planning for something positive in the near future, and then despite your attempts at sabotage I do my best to ensure that this hope becomes a reality. You know that you cause me great frustration. Alongside this, I realise that some things I used to do I can no longer, and others I did more easily are now harder. Don't think smugly of this, as there are also many things which previously I would have avoided or struggled with that I now tackle with relish and confidence, as witnessed in my diary entries.

I am not fooled by your attempt at a benign appearance when you take me into the shadows, and I know from the experience of the last two or three years that the challenges you set before me are both within and without. Despite early acceptance I understand I cannot shake off your clutches as you grip me closer to you, but with help and support I am being empowered to better deal with the anxiety you engender and encourage. Some have emerged to take my hand and lead me from the fog into the sun, and it is with them I will go forward. Many of these good people are by my side as I walk and talk, and this is evidenced in my new book *Walk the Walk, Talk the Talk*. Who would have thought that, when I was told to 'call it a day' and resign from my master's course and then my job, a few years later instead of slouching in my armchair I would be sitting upright at my desk writing a book? A book which you know will challenge you, dementia, to the core of your existence.

You see, dementia, your knowledge of me is certainly esoteric. Did you realise that I have been written off before, first as a child born on the 'wrong side of the track', and surrounded by low expectations and doors which seemed to close more readily than open? Then as a teenager where signposts placed before me led only to blind alleys and cul de sacs with one exception, this being the 'yellow brick road' which for me led to my Oz – university, a place of truth, hope and positivity which I arrived at only through my own determination, drive, focus and desire to learn and teach. I am still on that road.

As I walk alone at times I am never really alone because on these occasions I always listen to music on my iPod. One piece which inspires me and helps me confront you has become almost my theme tune at talks I give. There are many threads in this song which I relate so closely to – read these words, 'dear dementia', and recognise the ME in your name – deMEntia – because whilst I am here I will do everything I can to keep one step ahead of you and stay on the sunlit road rather than join you by the wayside in the fog.

'While I Am Here' by Eric Bogle

While I am here
I will make to you a promise from this simple man
That whatever I may do, I'll do the best I can
I will try to make a song that touches someone's heart
Though I may not do it all but I will make a start
Don't know how long I can stay, but I'll do all that I can while I am here

While I am here, I have dues I have to pay
Only once to pass this way
This is my promise for the days
While I am here

While I am here
I will recognise that weakness is my constant friend

I'll keep it to myself except for now and then
I will not become a shadow of my present self
A watcher with no words to offer someone else
Don't know how long I can stay, but I'll do all that I can
While I am here

A million miles may lie between the man I'd like to be
And how I live my life from day to day
I'll take my chance, make my choice and look again to see
A million miles is just one step away

While I am here
I will always seek to love and be loved in return
I will never raise my hand, and never point a gun
I'll not spend too much time thinking of when I'll go
Leave it better than I found it, though no one may ever know
Don't know how long I can stay but I'll do all that I can
While I am here

While I am here
I have dues I have to pay
Only once I have to pass this way
This is my promise for the days
While I am here

From the album *Other People's Children* by Eric Bogle and
reproduced with permission of John Munro and Eric Bogle

I have no suit of armour against you, no immunity, no tricks, but what
I do have are WORDS, HOPE and SPIRIT, and those I will hold on to for
as long as I possibly can – maybe forever.

Yours defiantly

Keith

2017
—
'Flowering'

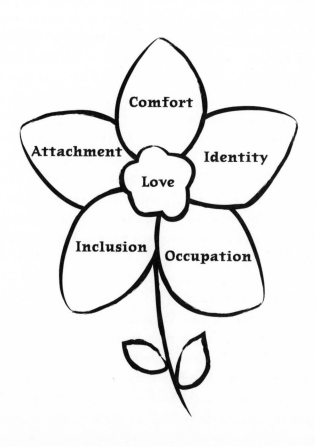

4th January – Canterbury

Today saw the satisfying result of six days sorting dementia files, tidying up and reorganising my office. This has needed doing for some time as I have been hoarding lots of papers. I hate throwing things away normally but there are times when I need to. The office now looks neat and tidy, everything is much more orderly, so hopefully I can find things more easily. I filled five dustbin bags which we'll take to the tip or shred. I felt comfortable and contented, so now I'm able to sit down and think about writing, and came up with this...

> 'Today is going to be different, different from yesterday, different from last week and different from tomorrow. Today is going to be a sunny day and, as I feel well, the words that sometimes slip through the crevices in my mind will be forthcoming. I am alone and yet I am with friends, friends who I sense are sitting by my side, smiling, encouraging, suggesting, prompting, affirming and bringing warmth to what yesterday was a chilled breeze. I want to write. I need to write. I feel the desire to put into words my deepest thoughts whilst I still retain the ability to do so. So, I write.'

10th January – Canterbury

I'm feeling more confident now in engaging in teleconferences, as evidenced by seeking to establish ideas and suggestions with Matt Murray, Hilary Doxford, Chris Roberts and myself about the 3 Nations Dementia Working Group. The group has big ambitions and aims, and I'm thrilled to have been brought in by the group, who have already started the ball rolling. They did this by examining the Scottish Working Group and others internationally.

12th January – Canterbury

When I read an engaging book, I'm always sad to reach the end, and I felt that today in coming to the close of *Dadland*. I really loved it. The book focuses upon the story of a man who bravely served in the war as an undercover agent in both Europe and the Far East, and later developed dementia. One strength of the book was the way it examined family relationships through the words of the author, his daughter Keggie Carew.

Speaking of books, this evening I should have gone to the Canterbury

Book Club to speak about *Walk the Walk, Talk the Talk*. Unfortunately, by 7 p.m. there was a heavy snowfall, which necessitated the cancelling of the session. It's the only snow we've had so far this winter, and I feel frustrated and disappointed that it resulted in the cancelling of an event I was looking forward to. Hopefully an alternative date will be found before too long. As I look out the window, there's a blanket of white, so the decision to cancel was the right one to make. Almost simultaneously, both mine and Rosemary's minds were transported back ten years to when each winter I would have to make an early-morning decision on whether to open the school on days when snow fell heavily.

15th January – Canterbury

I'm staggered that the YouTube film *Keith Oliver's Story* has now past 25,000 views and seems to be attracting on average just over 120 a week. There are now people writing comments alongside the film, and having taught myself how to respond I am engaging in writing replies to people who have taken the trouble to write.

19th January – London

Rosemary and I attended the regular Young Onset Dementia workstream meeting at Waterloo. Today we were able to discuss the third draft of the GP guide that we're working on as a group, which is really beginning to take shape now. Linked to our attempts to reach and engage better with GPs, I was able to tell the group about an article featuring my story which has just been published in the *British Medical Journal*. I feel privileged and honoured to have been able to fulfil this because I sense that the readers of the journal are professionals who may derive some benefit from reading stories such as mine.

20th January – Canterbury

For the first time in over five years, KMPT invited me to St Martin's Hospital today to sit on an interview panel seeking to appoint a psychologist to the local team. There were two psychologists and myself on the panel and two candidates, one of whom, Jo, was successful in the interview and will be a very good addition to the team. I felt comfortable in my role on the panel and was able to ask questions, and my opinion of the candidates was considered along with those of the two professionals sitting alongside me.

24th January – Canterbury

Following a therapy session with Yvette three weeks ago, today was the 20th of the 20 that were originally commissioned by the Trust to support me. Yvette and I decided it would be helpful to continue for another set of ten, but there will be no more beyond that. Thanks to Yvette I've felt a re-emergence of a positive, constructive inner voice, alongside the realisation of the increased challenges that dementia poses for me.

26th January – London

Today should have marked the launch of the Dementia Pathways document that resulted from the ABA expert research group that Lewis supported me on over the past year. I was asked to speak at the launch, which was held at the Royal College of Psychiatrists. The conference was a good one, and the speakers spoke very eloquently about the pathway and about how important the document will be in helping steer dementia care forward over the next few years. The only downside was that the document wasn't ready to hand out to people. There clearly are some issues around some elements of the pathway which still need to be resolved. This was very puzzling and disappointing.

27th January – Canterbury

Felt dementia got the better of me today. Thick fog descended. Not sure why and not sure what to do about it, other than to rest up for the day, take stock and move on tomorrow.

1st February – Sittingbourne

With Lewis's support I attended the initial meeting of a service user group which has been established by Jocelyne and Lewis in Sittingbourne to mirror the work that groups such as the Forget Me Nots are doing. This forms part of our desire to increase service user involvement within KMPT. I know Jocelyne is absolutely committed to this, and in the assistant psychologist Lewis, and Polly the placement student, she has two very able lieutenants.

My role at this inaugural meeting alongside Chris Norris was to outline our experience and to encourage the group to do lots of things which will benefit their wellbeing and improve services in that area. This now gives us a fourth Kent group alongside the Forget Me Nots, Memorabilia in Maidstone and the Sunshiners in Dover.

2nd February – Canterbury

Rosemary and I visited Charles and Pauline Ryan at their home in Canterbury today. Charles is a retired member of the Forget Me Nots and was a fellow *Welcome to Our World* author, an ex-barrister with some amazing stories to tell. It's such a shame that his dementia has resulted in him needing to retire from the Forget Me Nots. One subject we discussed was the excellent support Rosemary and Pauline, like many others, receive from Sinead, the Admiral Nurse for our area who meets with them as a carer to chat about how things are for them. Although we could certainly use more Admiral Nurses, currently Kent is better provided for than many parts of the country. In my view *all* carers should have access to an Admiral Nurse if they require this. I read recently that the number of these 'angels' has increased from 102 in the UK in 2012 to 140 in 2014, with an aim to exceed 200 as soon as possible in 2017. This is progress, but still nowhere near enough, especially when compared to the provision of Macmillan Nurses.

3rd February – London

After some considerable planning and discussions, today was the inaugural meeting of the steering group for the 3 Nations Dementia Working Group. The meeting was led by Matt Murray, and Hilary Doxford was elected as chair. There are 12 members of the steering group, most of whom were able to attend today or join us via the telephone. This represents one member from each Alzheimer's Society region. The meeting focused upon introductions, although many of us already knew each other, outlining what the key aims for the group are and then confirming them. The aims are largely about forming a go-to group for both the Alzheimer's Society and outside agencies, and in turn to be a critical friend to the society.

8th February – Godmersham

Reinhard, Chris Norris and I attended the launch of the Canterbury and Ashford Dementia Action Alliance in Godmersham near Canterbury, which was followed by a very pleasant lunch at a café in Chilham nearby.

This local event was useful in drawing together interested agencies in our region and provided a good platform for networking.

9th February – London

Because Reinhard was unable to attend today's DAA board meeting, Jocelyne came with me instead. Whilst I missed the conversations with Reinhard, it was lovely to be supported by Jocelyne, and we had a really useful day together discussing the DAA meeting and beyond. The board has now been redefined as a steering group, which is a subtle though significant difference in the role of the group. Today we focused upon areas steering a pathway forward regarding the hospital campaign to make hospital stays more positive for people with dementia, and updating people on the Dementia Statements, alongside seeing a potential launch for a new campaign which will focus on seldom-heard groups. All interesting subjects I was able to engage with due to the preparation Jocelyne and I had made on the train up to London and her considerate support during the meeting.

Jocelyne and I also discussed on the journey the power of labelling people, especially negatively. After a professional life in which I had often to deal with the implications for children of being harshly or negatively labelled by staff, parents and peers, I am well placed to see the potential hazards. I, like many, hate the label of 'sufferer' as there is nothing constructive one can take from this; 'service user' is so impersonal and medical-speak; 'person affected with dementia' is helpful but is unclear as to how the person is affected – whether they or a loved one have the diagnosis; 'carer' is useful, and in many cases accurate, but does imply 'one-way traffic' of care which is not the case, and also, because many people who see themselves as carers are going to lose their loved one in the end to dementia, this can cause compounded grief and feelings of failure and guilt towards themselves; 'dementia journey' is a poor cliché – journeys should be fun and exciting: no one wants to go on this one-way trip. For me, 'person living with dementia' and the person's name, as shown in the story a while ago with Lewis (29th April 2013), are the best labels one can use for myself; in the case of Rosemary, 'wife' and 'supporter' are roles and labels which we are both very comfortable with.

13th February – London

Back to Devon House today for an Alzheimer's Society research panel meeting, supported by Polly, and afterwards we were joined by Jess. It was lovely to catch up with her, albeit briefly.

The panel meeting, as always, tabled an increasingly large amount of applications for care and wellbeing projects, and one notices the quality and the quantity of applications is increasing. Consequently, deciding what can be funded by the society is becoming increasingly more problematic, but this is a good problem to have. A number of recommendations for six or seven projects that could go ahead have now been placed with the board who meet next week.

14th February – Canterbury

Having completed the first 20 sessions with Yvette, today marked the first of the final ten. On the way to see her, as always, I had music on my iPod and I was reminded of a quote I saw recently from the Greek philosopher Plato who wisely stated: 'Music gives a soul to the universe, wings to the mind, flight to the imagination and life to everything.' I couldn't have said it better myself. I would agree with all of what the great man said.

That quote and the music inspired me to be relaxed in my session with Yvette, and areas that we talked about included writing a compassionate letter to myself, my childhood, the activities I'm engaged with connected to my envoy and ambassador role, and what my strengths are. She highlighted kindness, companionship and being non-judgemental. She said that I need to prepare myself better mentally beforehand for these sessions. I thought that listening to music was sufficient, but she felt I needed to get into a more relaxed frame of mind and to make more use of the app that she pointed me towards a while ago. Also I am to consider even more the issue of compassion towards myself. Using these ideas, Yvette suggested I write this letter to myself and to bring it to the next session, and to read it aloud to myself beforehand when preparing for the session.

16th February – Maidstone

Reinhard and I travelled up to Maidstone and were met by Chris Norris before going into an envoy meeting with Vincent Badu, who is one of the newly appointed directors at KMPT. We spoke for over an hour with Vincent, which was a lot of talking. It now remains to be seen what follows, particularly what comes from the Trust to support Chris and me in our role as envoys. There was some suggestion that we may be able to sit on an interview panel for the coming appointment for a senior post within the Trust.

21st February – Westgate-on-Sea

Rather than all of us having to travel up to London for the Young Onset Dementia workstream meeting, today we conducted a teleconference on the GP guide, which is coming together. Again, my confidence in this way of communicating is improving, and I engaged in today's teleconference at James's flat at Westgate. The amount of preparation and support I had before helps me enormously.

22nd February – Canterbury

DEEP called a special meeting at Canterbury's Marlowe Theatre for members of the Forget Me Nots group to provide feedback on the theatre and how dementia friendly it is or could be. Philly Hare came down from York to lead the meeting and it will form part of DEEP's work on dementia-friendly public places and facilities. Our theatre is relatively new, being reopened after a rebuild five years ago. Some of our ideas and suggestions are either too expensive or simply not possible to put into place, but had they been sought five or six years ago then they could have been implemented more easily and cheaply then. Some suggestions revolve around the decoration of the theatre and the entrance and some around the seating. A few things which could be addressed relatively cheaply include signage, making the entrance more easily identifiable and placing seat numbers on the seats where they can be clearly seen.

27th February – London

Following on from the Alzheimer's Society research panel meeting two weeks ago, today one of the placement students, Celina, supported me in attending the follow-up board meeting. It was my turn, which comes around once every two years, to attend, and I was asked to speak on behalf of four applications, which I did as honestly and comprehensively as I could. Some I spoke more strongly in favour of than others, but the idea is to present to the board the views of the panel and to enhance and elaborate some of those comments with views of my own.

28th February – Oxford

Reinhard, Rosemary and I were invited by Jane Fossey, a clinical psychologist based in Oxford, and Larry Gardiner, a person with dementia, to come over and speak at an Oxford NHS event. The event was very well supported and provided some informative sessions from local people. Our role was to illustrate the work that's happening in Kent, and perhaps how Oxford can benefit and draw from our experience. One aspect of the day was that there was an artist recording the event on a giant sheet of paper as a cartoon representation. This I found particularly fascinating.

2nd–26th March – Adelaide, Australia

Although we missed out travelling to Australia last year, this year Rosemary and I were able to spend three weeks in our beloved Adelaide. This is our 17th visit, our seventh since the day on 2010 when advised by my neurologist to cancel the visit which we had planned for that year. Whilst long-distance travel has got more challenging for us, the support we get from Vicky and previously Eva and Misty at the flight centre is outstanding and essential. We have for some time had Meet and Assist at the various airports and extra help with our booking arrangements. In addition we now base ourselves in a wonderful apartment by the beach entitled Seawall. The people there are so friendly and the apartment is wonderful, plus being so convenient for all that Glenelg, Adelaide's prime seaside suburb, has to offer. Friends who previously we would have stayed with or visited now kindly come and visit us, either at the apartment or at cafés nearby. Whilst this illustrates a change in our needs, it also shows how we can still sustain what for us is a wonderful experience.

People back home in England would, I'm sure, find it strange that whilst they're fleeing from the freezing cold in early March we are at the same time seeking shelter from the heat in Australia. Today is one such day. The mercury by noon had rocketed to 42 degrees Celsius, prompting our decision to seek sanctuary from the sun and head off in a – thankfully – air-conditioned bus to the mall and cinema. Once the bus eased into the terminus and the electronic door gasped and opened, we ventured out into the heat. Fortunately, it was a short walk to the mall and cinema. Unsurprisingly it was clear that many others had the same thought as us.

For the rest of our time 'down under' the sun shone but the temperature was maintained at around the 30–35 mark, which allowed us to indulge in our annual regular swims in the beautifully tranquil ocean which now enticingly awaits us two minutes' stroll from our apartment.

29th March – Canterbury

Yvette has asked me to write a compassionate letter to myself and to bring it in today to the therapy session with her. She insisted that I read it aloud to her, which helped both of us to gain a greater understanding of the letter. Here is the letter:

Dear Keith

I've been wanting to write to you for some time, and following a prompt from a mutual friend, I feel the time is right to express some thoughts which I hope you will find helpful.

I feel I've known you for a very long time, indeed for most or all of your life, and whilst I am sure that the last few years have been very challenging I know you well enough to realise that the Keith I and others really know does still remain. For some people, showing sincerity, compassion and thoughtful kind words and actions towards others is hard. In your case, through your personality and experience, these come more easily. Conversely, you have at times resisted and not recognised the need to be the recipient, but this should now change. I've mentioned knowing you since your childhood, seeing you as a sensitive, quiet, single child who did quite well at school whilst enjoying the company of a range of friends.

You always came to the aid of others, at times stepping in when you thought this was required, thinking you could help someone who needed help. I wonder if others did the same for you. I think you have not always sought from others what you readily gave to them. Now is the time to refill some of your reservoir of compassion.

I know that at times you have felt let down. Maybe this is true. But at others, watching on, I can say that this has not always been the case, but has been your perception of the situation. I recognise that adjusting to seeing the world through different eyes can be difficult for anyone, including you, but do continue to seek the positives within the challenges you're facing at the time.

Do carry on thinking about the positives, around what you describe as the balance scales between the cognitive and the emotional aspects of engagement with others and the way you see yourself. I'm not going to patronise you or minimise your very real fears by saying don't be scared, but do try and draw on your inner strength from your innate ability to manage this.

Only you and I know how it is for you. You conceal the inner impact of your difficulties with a mask and the coping strategies that you have, and are continuing to develop, which will help protect you and enable you to remain connected to others. Consequently, there are times when people don't know what to look for, or what to ask in order to help you. You and I know this is especially the case when dementia makes the most mischief. Please take from this letter the key message to live in the moment, to not to judge yourself too harshly and to try to see in yourself the Keith who is seen by others, both close to you and those who pass by briefly. Use the strategies that have served you well in the past allied to those which might be new to you, which others who really care have offered, for in that way you have an even greater chance of living as well as possible.

Until next time, goodbye

Myself

When I got home that evening, I put on my computer and was uplifted to see that recently the Alzheimer's Society had very generously made *Walk the Walk, Talk the Talk* their choice for World Book Day. Maybe the letter is starting to have a positive impact.

30th March – St Albans

Alongside speaking at the unveiling of Abbeyfield's award-winning garden at Hampton Court Flower Show and at their annual conference, today gave

Rosemary and me the opportunity to visit their headquarters. It was the first time I'd been to the historic city of St Albans. Part of our visit was spent at Abbeyfield's headquarters recording an interview about my life and living with dementia for inclusion on their website and on YouTube, and part of the day was spent exploring the historic city and cathedral.

31st March – Canterbury

With Sammi's support I was able to attend a meeting today with Pat Chung at Canterbury Christ Church University to discuss an occupational therapy project, which is funded by the College of Occupational Therapists, to explore the benefits and the impacts that the Kent Enablement Service has on people living with dementia.

4th April – London

Rosemary and I were thrilled and honoured to be able to attend and speak at an all-party parliamentary group event at the House of Lords, seeking to explain the potential benefits of engaging with the arts for mental health. Within the group attending there was a very diverse range of people. The discussion was observed and recorded by famous artist David Shrigley, whose most famous piece of work, entitled 'Really Good', currently stands on the plinth in Trafalgar Square. We had lunch with David, during which time we discussed a range of topics, including football, and I was delighted to hear he's a Nottingham Forest supporter.

This prompted me to show him a copy of *Walk the Walk, Talk the Talk*, pointing out the chapter in there about Forest. He promptly bought the book and asked if I had written anything else. Coincidentally I happened to have a copy of *Welcome to Our World* in my bag and he was keen to buy that as well.

After lunch it was back into the meeting. The range of people involved included ex-soldiers, ex-prisoners and ex-drug addicts, all of whom had confronted severe mental health issues, but had utilised the creative arts to help them to live as well as possible. The conclusion to the day was a filmed interview between myself and Lord Howarth, who was chairing the project. He was interested to know about my life with dementia and how I use arts to help me (by way of writing). I told him the story of the circle dance (see 13th–14th July 2011) and how much benefit that provided me with at the time.

5th April – London

As always, Rosemary and I (or whoever is supporting me) travel up to London on the high-speed train, which travels from Canterbury West to St Pancras in 50–55 minutes. This is a real asset to have. Alongside this, often the meetings are in the area between St Pancras, Euston or Kings Cross, and today was an example of that. Rosemary and I walked from St Pancras to a meeting held at the Wellcome Foundation. The event was a consensus event, seeking to change the 'I' Statements that formed the basis of the National Dementia Declaration to a set of new Dementia Statements. The event was facilitated by the Alzheimer's Society with an external chair. A series of lively discussions took place, both as a whole group and through small round tables. Our group discussion was supported by Elizabeth Oliver from the Alzheimer's Society. At the end of today I was delighted that the Dementia Statements have now been rewritten as the following, which will be unveiled later this year...

We have the right to be recognised as who we are, to make choices about our lives including taking risks and to contribute to society. Our diagnosis should not define us, nor should we be ashamed of it.

We have the right to continue with day-to-day and family life without discrimination or unfair cost, to be accepted and included in our communities and not live in isolation or loneliness.

We have the right to an early and accurate diagnosis and to receive evidence-based, appropriate, compassionate and properly funded care and treatment from trained people who understand us and how dementia affects us. This must meet our needs wherever we live.

We have the right to be respected and recognised as partners in care, provided with education, support services and training which enables us to plan and make decisions about the future.

Finally, we have the right to know about and decide if we want to be involved in research that looks at cause, cure or care for dementia and be supported to take part.

I, like everyone else in the room, was delighted by the compromises, discussions and the involvement of everybody at the event which resulted in the wording of those statements. Now it's a case of getting them out there and being effectively used.

6th April – Canterbury

For Christmas, Rosemary and I once again had Marlowe Theatre vouchers from our son Gareth and family. We utilised them today to go and see *Sunny Afternoon*, which is basically the Kinks story. I love their music, especially the pieces from the 1960s, and one song which often worms into my mind when walking across Westminster Bridge in London is Waterloo Sunset. It's in my mind as I'm writing this diary entry.

7th April – Canterbury

A very different perspective today of being in the same room at the same time with Yvette because today I helped her with interviewing for a placement student from Canterbury Christ Church University, who was seeking to join next year's cohort. The student's name is Abi, and she came over very positively. Both Yvette and I are absolutely convinced that she will be a good addition to the student group next year. What I found particularly interesting, along with her engaging and pleasant personality, was the fact that she attended the Brit School in Croydon, one that Adele and many other famous names have attended, including Jessie J and Amy Winehouse. I believe she studied theatre there and was also involved with singing and dancing. The module that she studied was called 'Community Arts', so I hope that when she begins her placement she and I get the chance to talk about some aspects of the arts.

11th April – London

Whilst it was a big loss when Lisa left the Alzheimer's Society, and I do miss working with her on the service user workshops, today marked a new chapter in the sense that her replacement, Elizabeth Oliver (I sat on her interview panel also), delivered her first workshop with me supporting. It was actually quite seamless between working with Lisa and working with Elizabeth, and consequently I enjoyed working with Elizabeth today. After the workshop, during which I was ably supported by Kristina (one of this year's students), I met with Lawrence Ivil, who until recently had been alongside Paul Miles leading the Dementia Diaries project. Lawrence now has returned to university for further study, and I wanted to meet to get him to sign my copy of *Walk the Walk, Talk the Talk*, which I am trying to get all friends who contributed to do.

12th April – Canterbury

For some time now, in fact since 2011, eight of us have met monthly between September and April, originally as part of a U3A family history group, but now as friends, to discuss family history and the world and life in general. Today was the last of these meetings until the summer break, although we do plan as previously to have a summer lunch together. Consequently, I felt upbeat at the end of this meeting and very relaxed and positive, which set me in a good frame of mind for being dropped off by Rosemary at St Martin's Hospital for my periodic appointment with Richard Brown, which also went well.

19th April – London

Rosemary joined me in a meeting which focused upon innovation at the quarterly Dementia Action Alliance meeting with the College of Occupational Therapists. The day was chaired by Neil Mapes from Dementia Adventure alongside Chris and Jayne Roberts. Presentations included looking at how the NHS can be more innovative, and how it can utilise private initiatives alongside in-house programmes. There was also a good opportunity for members to share initiatives that they're embarking on, and one that I sat in on was from Alzheimer's Research UK, which looked at introducing a virtual reality app. Not for me, but interesting to see what was available.

What I did find more worthwhile were presentations by Dawn Brooker about a project that is currently being run out in Worcestershire, focused upon the community-based hubs helping people to adjust to life with dementia and giving people time and space to discuss their condition. Following that I attended a session by Wayne Goddard, a commissioner from Doncaster, who I know from the ABA ERG piece of work. Wayne spoke about innovative approaches to commissioning work in Doncaster, some of which revolved around a different use of the Admiral Nursing Service.

25th April – London

I'm delighted to bring Rosemary into the Reading Well project at The Reading Agency. Previously I'd been supported by Tricia Fincher from Kent Libraries who has now retired, and I'm not sure her replacement has quite the same level of commitment and time to devote to the project and working alongside me. It's lovely to get Rosemary involved in this project, which is seeking to involve older people who are lonely and isolated in the use of books and through reading friends to become happier and more connected. At the end Rosemary and I went for a coffee with Nada, who is also part of this project, which gave us a very pleasant closure to the day.

27th April – Dover

Through Jean, our friend in Shepherdswell, I'd been invited to go and speak at the Dover Senior Citizen's Forum about dementia and my experience of living with it. Bearing in mind that most of the audience were over the age of 70, it did present a certain challenge in getting the balance right in terms of giving the people in the audience the facts and telling them what my experience has been without engendering or building upon fears they already held. I gave the talk, it went well, and the response from the audience was extremely positive. At the end I had the opportunity to sell my book *Walk the Walk, Talk the Talk*, and every copy of the book that I took sold. There was also a raffle, and it was lovely that the main prize was a bottle of gin; I walked away with that as well. All in all a very good day.

28th April – Chatham

Although I've been to the University of Kent at the Medway site, this was the first time that I'd been to the Canterbury Christ Church Medway site since 2011 when I was there with Penny Hibberd. I went today with Pat Chung and Sammi, one of this year's students, and gave a very similar talk to the one that I delivered to the Canterbury students. Again, the response was very positive and similar to that from the Canterbury cohort, but what was different was the composition of the student group. This particular group was much more diverse in age and ethnic background.

4th May – London

Following the recent teleconference for the Young Onset Dementia workstream, focusing on the GP guide, today was our next face-to-face meeting where we built upon the discussion conducted in the teleconference. We are now at the point where we're ready to share the guide with the full steering group. After the meeting in Waterloo, Rosemary and I met up with Mycal Miller at St Pancras for a coffee and discussed with him a proposed course that he wishes to undertake at one of the London universities and which he's asked me to act as a referee, which of course I am delighted to do. The film that Mycal and I made back in 2012 is still one of the pieces of work that I'm most proud of and, as previously noted in the diary, continues to grow in number of YouTube views by approximately 120 a week; this is great credit to his professionalism.

8th May – Canterbury and Oxford

After a SURP meeting in Canterbury led by Kate Comfort, I left early and met Rosemary before heading off to Oxford by train because tomorrow we are due to sit on an interview panel seeking to appoint a new Young Dementia UK manager for the national network. The post is entitled 'national development manager'. By heading off early, we were able to spend a bit of time today in Oxford as tourists. I was keen to encourage Rosemary to follow up a conversation I'd had with Eric Harmer recently, linked to a shared interest in C.S. Lewis. Eric had encouraged me to go and visit the Eagle and Child pub in Oxford, and Rosemary and I were able to do that this afternoon. Very quaint, old-fashioned pub where you could sense the presence of people like Lewis and Tolkien in its poky snug-type rooms. In the evening we were able to stay in a very pleasant hotel in the outskirts of the city where tomorrow the interview will be conducted. I took with me the seven letters of application and application forms that I'd been sent by Tessa from Young Dementia UK to read once again. There are some very good candidates to be interviewed tomorrow. The job advert attracted 108 applicants, so I didn't envy the professionals who narrowed it down to the seven that we are going to meet. I'm very much looking forward to that.

9th May – Oxford

Interviewing seven candidates in a day was a challenge, but I'm delighted that a successful applicant emerged, and Donna Chadwick will be offered the job. Donna came over brilliantly in the interview and will, I'm sure, admirably fill the very big hole left by Sarah Plummer.

10th May – Canterbury

In a sense today's appointment with Yvette, which is the 24th of the 30, sits alongside one that took place two weeks ago. The area of focus that we've concentrated on in these two appointments is the construction of something called 'My Self-Compassion Care Plan'. This plan should sit alongside the care plan which was written by Richard, my consultant, and me, and which took me four years to get and ten minutes for Richard and me to co-produce. This Self-Compassion Care Plan required more thinking on my part and more time. It covers key issues that I confront each day, part of which is my fear of letting people down and losing contact with folk, the difficulty I experience in my own company when not busy, my occasional reticence in asking help from others and how I sense my world is physically shrinking. Alongside these is difficulties with time management and losing track of time.

Yvette, both today and on 26th April, patiently talked me through these areas and alongside that tried to give me suggestions for better dealing with those difficulties. With regard to the fear of letting people down and losing contact, often I worry that people will think ill of me and desert me. The consequence of this is that I'm puzzled and confused as I don't usually remember what has been said, but do remember how the action made me feel. There is something in trying to please others which is new to me as I used to seek respect and not necessarily being liked.

Sometimes I feel I've lost some sense of self-respect and self-esteem. I need to recognise that it's not possible to be liked all the time, and to savour and enjoy this when it happens, then try and retain this sense of the moment and not seek for its repeat or extension. Quiet days are hard, and evenings when the TV cannot capture my interest are very difficult. Rosemary and I are playing card games and board games in the evening to help keep us both alert and our minds on something constructive. It is difficult because both of us get tired as well. When the better weather comes, and hopefully there'll be more of that soon, we both love sitting in the garden with a cup of tea and a biscuit, admiring the view and watching the world go by. Occasionally the idea of doing that on my own seems to be a good idea as well.

Being aware of not being too hard on myself is important and I get frustrated that I can't do what I used to do so easily, but then I do try to balance that by celebrating new skills, such as writing and swimming – both of which I did before, but not as well as I think I do now.

11th May – London

Five minutes outside Canterbury West station our high-speed train ground to a halt at a level crossing near to where we live. After a short time it was clear from some activity outside the train that there was a problem. Sadly, a young man had done what tragically too many seem to do these days, which is to throw himself in front of a train to commit suicide. The train manager was great and kept us as informed as he possibly could, and whilst Rosemary and I felt for the young man we also felt great sympathy for the driver and train manager who had to witness and deal with the situation. We did eventually make it to London for our meeting at the Alzheimer's Society, three hours late.

16th May – London

Dementia Action Alliance board meeting attended with Reinhard, where we looked at confirming the Dementia Statements as they were written recently at the consensus event we attended at the Wellcome Foundation. Confirming discussions went smoothly, as did the work around the Seldom Heard Groups call to action (From Seldom Heard to Seen and Heard), and the desire to focus upon specific groups within the community, these being primarily the prison population and the LGBT community.

17th–19th May – London

Some years ago I attended SATs training for Key Stage 2 science markers at the Connaught Rooms in West London and it was a thrill to be able to take Rosemary there today to attend the Alzheimer's Society conference being held at this prestigious venue. We didn't stay there overnight, staying instead at a local Travelodge, which served our purposes well. On the 17th we met with Matt Murray to plan our co-presented talk which is planned for the 18th. The topic we are talking about is focusing on co-production in the service user professional roles at the Alzheimer's Society, and looking at the programme there's a fascinating menu of talks by researchers which I'm looking forward to.

This next entry is made on 19th May and now I'm looking back on the last two days: the talk that Matt and I delivered went down very well and I enjoyed co-presenting with him as well as co-producing what we were saying. The process has been a good one, through planning to delivery. Also, amongst the fascinating array of talks given by researchers was one by a researcher from Durham University who explained to us how the amygdala works in connection with the emotional and cognitive balance within the brain, and this for me was the first time I'd had explained what I experience frequently.

Another interesting session was one with Doug Brown, the director of research at the Alzheimer's Society, when Peter Mittler, an eminent person with dementia who is a retired professor from Manchester University and human rights expert, and I questioned Doug on the care element of the research programme at the forthcoming dementia research institute.

The conference also gave a platform for the launch of the 3 Nations Dementia Working Group alongside the Dementia Statements, and this was conducted on stage by way of an interview led by Bill Turnbull from the BBC. Five people with dementia, including myself, sat on a red settee (it felt like *BBC Breakfast*) with Bill asking us each to speak about one of the statements. I was asked to speak about the fourth statement, which focuses on the right to be respected and recognised as partners in care, provided with education, support, services and training which enables us to plan and make decisions about the future. For me they are all important, but with my background in education it was felt that this was possibly the most appropriate one for me to address.

22nd May – Canterbury

Tree of Life workshop at Thanington, led by Elizabeth Field and supported by assistant psychologists Lucy and Becca. Five Forget Me Nots and two

Sunshiners attended. I had a lovely, 'sunny' day despite the fact that it didn't begin in this way and I nearly didn't go – I am so pleased that I did, and it was down to the three staff leading and my compatriots present that I was led from the fog into the sun. The workshop is designed to help people focus upon their strengths and to see themselves aligned to family and friends, both through giving and receiving support. During the course of the day, using a template of a large tree we each constructed a visual representation of ourselves where the roots are your background; the ground is where you currently see yourself in life; the trunk, which is the part I found the hardest, is your strengths, skills and abilities; branches illustrate your hopes, wishes, goals and dreams; the leaves are important people in your life; fruits are given by others; and flowers are fruits you give to other people. We didn't have time for the concluding element – the seeds, which are things you wish to leave behind, possibly by way of a legacy.

Through the patient support available to me I was so pleased with my final tree and felt keen to share and support the efforts of others taking part. This was mutual; when we were invited to describe another person by writing one or two words on their tree, one friend, for whom English is her second language, wrote on my tree 'driveness' and 'kindness'. I'll take that, thank you.

The conclusion to the workshop involved us sharing our completed trees, placing them together to represent a forest, using the metaphor that trees, like people, function better collectively; we then discussed what storms might threaten the trees and how these might be minimised. All in all a memorable day, which proved extremely positive in supporting me through difficult times and helping to restore and maintain my vulnerable self-confidence.

23rd May – London

It was with mixed feelings today that I attended a service user training workshop with placement student Celina. The mixed feelings were that the session went really well, with a very engaged and positive group, and that it was great to see Elizabeth Oliver's confidence growing in the role. The negative aspect was that it will be Elizabeth's last session, which is such a great pity as I really feel that we're getting to know each other and working well together. It appears that the role of engagement and participation officer for London isn't the one that fits her needs best, so she's going to return to her previous role in Sutton, working on the Vanguard project, and I wish her well in that future role.

1st June – London

Three Nations Dementia Working Group meeting at Crutched Friars with Rosemary. A full and varied agenda had been prepared beforehand and one senses the group is starting to get established, something which will be enhanced and will go forward once we are comfortable with the terms of the group and have an established project officer appointed to help steer and energise us all.

6th June – London

I really feel honoured to be a part of the Angela Project, which is seeking to improve the diagnosis pathway for people with young onset dementia and then to improve post-diagnostic support, both of which Rosemary and I feel passionately about. Today's meeting gave me reassurance that the work is moving forward effectively.

8th June – Canterbury

Lewis and I delivered a talk to four student volunteers connected with the Dreams and Visions project today. Liz came for the start of the session, did the introductions and set the scene for the project, then she left to collect her children from school. We were both well prepared, and Lewis had devoted a lot of time to constructing a substantial talk about dementia for the students. A pity only four turned up. This was down to confusion at the university around communication. However, the four who came did seem interested and hopefully will attend as volunteers for the project. I don't know whether today's general election had an impact on student numbers.

9th June – London

Attended the Alzheimer's Show in Olympia with Rosemary as I had been asked to speak about *Walk the Walk, Talk the Talk*, which gives me opportunities to tell the audience about the process of writing the book, dip into the content, and sell the book at the event. One extract from the book I chose to read was written by my friend Melvyn Brooks from the Forget

Me Nots. In his piece he wrote, 'Keith and I do not always see eye to eye on things but that is what good friendship is all about.' For me those are some of the wisest words in the book.

Alongside this, I began my talk with a bottle of Prosecco in my hand, given to me earlier by Rachel Niblock from DEEP, by saying how proud I was today to come from Canterbury, as following yesterday's general election, the city has elected a Labour MP. This is the first time since 1844 that a Conservative has been toppled from their lofty perch.

Later at the show I joined a question and answer panel on the stage, composed of Dr James Warner, Andrea Sutcliffe (Chief Inspector, Adult Social Care, CQC), David Reynolds (chief scientific officer from Alzheimer's Research UK), Tim McLachlan from the Alzheimer's Society and myself. The questions from a large and enthusiastic audience came thick and fast and were well shared between the panel. At the end I made my way to the DEEP table, where there was a queue of people waiting to buy my book, which I was glad to be able to sign and dedicate for them.

14th June – London

One thing I really applaud about today's Young Dementia Network meeting is the diligent way this group is seeking to advance the cause of younger people with dementia by a mix of innovative projects such as the GP guide, whilst allying itself to the existing work of others, such as the Angela Project on diagnosis and post-diagnostic support, the work on rights, the DAA Seldom Heard Groups call to action, and making the new Dementia Statements meaningful for younger people below the age of 65. As is now customary, afterwards Rosemary and I formed a part of what is now labelled by me as a 'debriefing group' in a local hostelry.

15th June – Canterbury

Moving forward with the Dreams and Visions project, I was able to meet today with Clive Richardson from Canterbury City Council to discuss which room may be able to be used by us at the Beaney and what the cost would be to be able to utilise this facility.

Following this, when I got home, I met with Reinhard to begin writing our joint presentation for the forthcoming Faculty of Psychology for Older People conference, which will be held in Durham. The talk we are seeking to deliver focuses on our professional friendship – how we met and have worked together over the past five years.

16th June – London

The six-monthly PREVENT monitoring meeting at the Middlesex Hospital, again supported by placement student Kristina. The benefit of having Kristina with me today was that she attended the previous meeting with me, plus the project conference held in the autumn. Consequently, Kristina is well informed, which enabled us to discuss the project both on the train and at the event, thus enabling us both to be fully involved at the meeting.

21st June – Canterbury

The 26th therapy session with Yvette. I came away from today feeling a sense of admiration for the way that Yvette is able to open me up and peel back the layers like that of an onion. We talked about not being judgemental of others, and in turn of ourselves. She recognises that I do judge people positively and not negatively, which is not always the case for some people.

One indication that summer is really with us is that the first lily burst into flower in our garden. Both Rosemary and I get so much pleasure from both working and sitting with a cup of coffee in our relatively small but vividly coloured garden amongst the flowers. So much is in bloom and there is still so much promise in what will emerge in weeks to come. This reminds me – a few days ago when weeding in a flower bed my mind was wandering as it often does these days. On this occasion I was thinking about friends and had the same thought that I had last summer – that friends are a bit like the beautiful flowers in our garden, they come into my life, enrich it and make me feel well and then fade – sometimes to return but sometimes just leaving the positive memory behind. I will cling onto this metaphor and I hope it will help me cope better with transient friendships.

23rd June–2nd July – Cornwall

Following our successful and enjoyable trip last year to St Agnes, Rosemary and I were keen to repeat this.

We stayed at the same cottage, which was as lovely as ever. Fortunately,

St Agnes has not changed over the past year, which is reassuring. The only difference between the holidays is that this year the weather wasn't as good, so whilst we were able to sunbathe on the Sunday and the Monday, the rest of the week had more rain than we would wish to see. Some days it was absolutely torrential. However, we had a good break and rest, so I feel my batteries are recharged and ready for future events that are in the pipeline. One potential project which has come out of the blue to land 'on my lap(top)' during our holiday was an email from Andrew James, senior commissioning editor at Jessica Kingsley Publishers. Andrew has invited me to meet and discuss with him a suggestion that I consider writing a book for them. This is, he says, partly initiated by my leadership of the *Welcome to Our World* book which he describes as 'intriguing'. I will follow this up once we return from holiday.

4th July – Canterbury

The Dreams and Visions project is moving forward. Liz and I met with Paul, the creative director at the Marlowe, who has now joined our team. We were able to explore the ways in which the theatre is able to support us; this could be by providing actors, Paul's time, and some sense of contacts that might prove fruitful as the project moves forward. Following this I stayed in Canterbury for one of the looked-forward-to monthly meetings I have with Eric and Jen. This was a little bit special as it marked the second anniversary of our first meeting and we duly celebrated with a cake!

5th–7th July – Swansea

My first visit to South Wales since I was a child, and Rosemary and I were honoured to be able to speak at the British Society of Gerontology's conference being held at Swansea University.

The platform I was asked to speak on was connected to the IDEAL project. It was a co-presentation with Catherine Quinn and Alex Hillman, and I was delighted to be able to speak about my involvement in the project.

We stayed at the Marriott Maritime which was a great location near the main beach. Because the weather was so glorious, Rosemary and I were able to supplement our time at the conference by strolling along the esplanade at the side of the hotel and admire the view looking out towards the Mumbles.

We were really quite taken by this, although the town of Swansea didn't hold any great attractions for us.

11th–14th July – Durham

Following the trip to Swansea, Rosemary and I were back on the train for a long trip, this time to Durham, where we were joined by Reinhard to present at the FPOP conference our talk about Reinhard and my six-year collaboration as professional friends.

I hadn't been to Durham since I'd been offered a teaching job there in 1977, and a couple of times to visit my university friends Terry and Liz, including being best man at their wedding in Durham in 1978.

The journey was a long one but very good, apart from the fact that Rosemary had a very concerning nosebleed on the train which lasted approximately an hour.

Alongside the conference, we enjoyed cordial social time with psychologists, many of whom we'd met previously. One leading professional who I had not previously met sat next to me for the conference dinner and introduced himself as a psychiatric nurse. Rosemary sensed he was more than this. It transpired that without realising it I was deep in conversation with Professor John Keady, whose books I have read in the past!

Mine and Reinhard's talk was well received. Whilst comfortable giving a solo talk I do actually much prefer those with a collaborator. At the end of the conference Rosemary and I enjoyed exploring the cathedral and strolling around the shops in the city.

18th–21st July – Windsor

Karon, our daughter, was keen for us to join her and William for his closing week as a pupil at Clewer Green First School where Karon is deputy head. William is now coming to the end of Year 4 and is about to transfer to a nearby middle school. During this week we were blessed to have the opportunity of watching his school play about Aladdin and the 40 thieves and to sit in on the leaver's service in nearby Clewer Church, then finally to attend the end-of-year assembly in the school hall, which brought back many happy memories of delivering those in my time at Blean and Barton. Alongside all of this, there was some wonderful family time spent with

Rosemary, Karon and William. Sadly, Nick wasn't able to join us because he is currently working abroad.

25th July – Canterbury

The focus for today's therapy session with Yvette was a quote that I'd picked up from a piece of literature, which was, 'The person isn't the problem, the problem is the problem.' I think this comes from a session of narrative therapy which Elizabeth Field delivered recently at the Durham conference. Yvette and I discussed this particular quote and the significance it has for my situation at the moment.

I was also able to update Yvette on the FPOP conference because she wasn't able to attend, and tell her about how positive I felt in delivering the collaboration with Reinhard. We also talked about issues around loyalty and what I consider this to mean, and how I cope when others are distressed. Yvette helped me to devise a plan for how to deal with this by way of what action to take, and how to respond through talking, listening, advising, eye contact and body language whilst maintaining a positive approach. All of which I was aware of and hope I have utilised in the past, but to be able to talk it through with her was as always very helpful.

We moved on then to talk about something I recorded as 'I care', not with the label of 'carer', but to always respond if a friend asks for help. I see this as a privilege. Also, the physicality of hugging for reassurance, and I was able to talk about my continued use of the mindfulness app, where I've been focusing on aspects of kindness and gratitude: being thankful, being hopeful, being appreciative.

Inspired and encouraged by talking it through with Yvette and last week with Reinhard, this afternoon I sent Andrew at Jessica Kingsley Publishers some suggestions for areas which might interest us regarding the potential new book. He responded immediately, and now the lines of communication are established we just need to see where they lead.

26th July – Chartwell

Whilst recognising the enormity of Churchill's efforts during World War II, I was most interested today in finding out more about his own mental health and his use of art to support his wellbeing. During our visit to his home near Sevenoaks with the Shepherdswell Wednesday Club, I spent time discussing this with one of the volunteer staff on duty and learnt a lot about the vulnerability of the great leader.

27th July – London

The ALWAYS group met today at Crutched Friars rather than its usual venue on the banks of Regent's Canal. The reason we did that was because James Pickett, head of research at the Alzheimer's Society, delivered an informative PowerPoint talk to the group about the initial findings that the IDEAL project is uncovering. This accompanied a discussion, led by Rachael Litherland. After the workshop, Rosemary and I travelled back to St Pancras, where we met Noel Collins, a consultant psychiatrist, to whom I had given some help with his book *The D-Word* by writing the introduction. To show his gratitude, Noel very kindly brought along some gifts and we had a lovely chat over a glass of wine at a venue outside St Pancras.

28th July – Canterbury

For the past few weeks several emails have been exchanged between Rachael Litherland, Philly Hare and ourselves to encourage us to travel to Geneva in order to present the documents written by the DEEP Think Tank on the rights of people with dementia. The UN Convention on the Rights of Persons with Disabilities (CRPD) is this year considering what the UK government are doing to meet the needs of those living with a range of disabilities, and DEEP have managed to secure a foothold for someone with dementia to attend and speak to the Convention and a rapporteur from the UN. I have been asked to fulfil this role, which with the support of Rosemary and Philly I am honoured to do, albeit with a great sense of nervousness. To add to my nerves, today was a frustrating day trying to achieve accreditation for the forthcoming trip to the UN. This proved very difficult, and despite some patient help from Philly Hare on the phone from York, it did provide some enormous challenges to us all which I believe we managed to overcome.

31st July – London

Following the Alzheimer's Society conference interchange between Doug Brown, Peter Mittler and myself, Doug kindly invited us to meet with him at Crutched Friars to discuss this in depth more privately. I thought it would be helpful to have Reinhard there too, so he kindly found time in his busy schedule to accompany me to the meeting, which gave him an opportunity to share his perspective on the project. Doug explored our views on care research and brought to the discussion a question around how we would feel about including technology in the care element at the dementia research institute. I expressed mixed feelings about this, recognising that technology is important to living well with dementia, but as a tool and not something that should take over, and certainly not to take over the human interaction which is of enormous benefit to people with dementia.

2nd August – Sittingbourne

Following an earlier visit to the newly established Sittingbourne service user group, now called 'Pathfinders', Lewis accompanied me again to join Jocelyne and the group in discussing the Dreams and Visions project and to see whether any of the group would wish to participate. It was lovely to spend time with them, but I'm not sure anyone in the group will be able to take part.

3rd August – Canterbury

Last night, with Chris Norris and Reinhard, I attended a meeting at Canterbury High School, entitled 'Exploring the strategic transformation plan for our local area'. This is an NHS initiative and we were asked to sit on a table marked 'Mental Health'. There was no one else there from the world of dementia, but there were people whose lives had been affected by other mental health issues, directly or through a family member. There were two or three presentations by senior consultants from the local acute hospitals, plus a presentation by the chief executive officer (CEO) of the East Kent Hospital Trust, who I fired questions at around the Trust's abilities to care for people with dementia in East Kent. At the end of the public meeting he came up to discuss this with me and invited me to email him to arrange a further 1:1 meeting, which I will do, and we'll see if anything further comes of that.

Also worth noting that today the YouTube film *Keith Oliver's Story* passed 30,000 views.

4th–9th August – Canterbury

Took four or five days off from my dementia roles to decorate the bathroom at home whilst Rosemary did the same in the en suite. All went reasonably well. I was pleased to be able to do this and to prove to myself that I was still able to wield a paintbrush and the results are very satisfying. The only negative was that the stool I was standing on to paint the coving collapsed, launching me into the bath below and causing me to crack two or three ribs, which resulted in an appointment at the GP for painkillers which I will begrudgingly take.

6th August – Canterbury

Just finished watching a repeat of *Countryfile* with James Wong visiting the Brecon Beacons to film daffodils growing, which in turn are being used to produce galantamine, the medication that I take each day.

10th August – London

Following Elizabeth Oliver's resignation as engagement and participation officer for London, today Rosemary and I attended the first of two days interviewing at Crutched Friars to secure a replacement. Also on the panel were Matt Murray and Sarah from the Alzheimer's Society. The post generated a good degree of interest with just over 20 applications. I was invited by Matt and Sarah to read what they thought were the best 11 and to help narrow them down to five, who we will interview today and next week.

16th August – Canterbury

My regular check-up with Richard Brown at St Martin's Hospital. Was it Leonardo da Vinci who wrote 'It's a poor teacher whose students do not surpass their master'? I have always held great aspirations for children I have taught and have said to them – aim for the stars and you might reach the moon. I tell audiences in conferences when this comes up that I used to care for Richard and now he cares for me. I hope and think that as a former pupil of mine from primary school days he recognises this.

17th August – London

Back up to Crutched Friars with Rosemary for day two of the interviews and I'm delighted to say we've managed to find a replacement for Elizabeth who looks very suitable. Her name is Sabrina and the verdict was unanimous. I look forward to working with her as I did with Elizabeth and Lisa previously.

18th August – Canterbury

The 28th therapy session with Yvette, at which we talked through my care plan. We talked about the homework, which was entitled 'I am a human being, hence I am important, no more no less'.

What Yvette wanted me to do was to look at how important I view myself in all the roles I occupy, not just the roles of envoy and ambassador. She was able to tell me about what she learns from the sessions as well, and she very kindly described me as 'inspiring', both my personality and what I'm seeking to achieve in life, which I found very moving and emotional.

20th August – Heathrow

On the high-speed train up to Heathrow today, in order to meet Philly Hare to connect with our flight to Geneva to speak at the United Nations, I was thrilled that a young lady sitting opposite on the train leant over and began by saying, 'Are you Mr Oliver?', which usually means it is an ex-pupil from Blean. It was an ex-pupil named Georgia, who told me that she was currently studying law at Hull. We happily chatted and she seemed extremely interested to hear that I was en route to the United Nations. This experience was similar to one which took place in Lloyds Bank a few days ago with Jasmine, who was about the same age as Georgia – in their early 20s – and was a former pupil of Blean school.

Having arrived at St Pancras, we met Philly at Kings Cross and boarded the Piccadilly Line for the long journey over to Heathrow. After a smooth check-in facilitated by Philly, we flew out on Swiss Air to Geneva.

Once in Geneva, we checked into a decent, quaint hotel situated near to the lake and the UN, chosen by Philly for its convenient location. In the warm Swiss sunshine we enjoyed an orientation stroll by the lake and talked about preparations for tomorrow's big day at the UN.

21st August – Geneva

Despite having spent a lot of time attempting to register online, the outcome of which was successful for Philly and myself, it appeared that it was unsuccessful for Rosemary. Getting through security at the UN this morning was very challenging for Rosemary and consequently for Philly and me, who wouldn't go through without her. Eventually a senior security officer did resolve the issue, but it took approximately an hour to do so.

Once successfully in the building we then made our way through the labyrinth of UN corridors to the room where I was to meet with the rapporteur connected to the CRPD. This meeting was very challenging. I thought he would present as a senior civil servant, in suit and tie like myself. The first shock was that he was in T-shirt and jeans and clearly severely disabled himself and confined to a wheelchair, with a number of aides to administer to his needs. He was Swedish and there were no gentle pleasantries by way of introductions. He threw in an opening 'grenade' by abruptly asking, 'So tell me why you consider yourself to be disabled?' I was caught off guard by this and felt that the 30-minute 'interrogation' by him was extremely challenging. I did my best to put the case of people with dementia in our country and the way our rights are not being best represented and upheld by our government. He did warm a little during the meeting but I was left drained, confused and upset by the experience. Philly did her best to reassure me that I had done as well as anyone could in the situation.

Following this, the three of us tried to settle and compose ourselves with a coffee before going through to the main UN auditorium where I would present the case for people with dementia to the international CRPD. Although nervous I felt much more at ease in this setting. The UK slot came near the end and dementia was at the end of this segment. I listened to a range of disability groups and individuals putting their case to the international committee, and then armed with my script I settled into what I think was a passionate, reasoned summary of the needs of those living with and affected by dementia – what is needed to ensure our rights are not trampled.

Alongside Alan Bennett's excellent book *Keeping On Keeping On*, I am currently also reading Tony Benn's diaries, which I am finding very insightful. Benn says that protest doesn't work but making demands does, and he uses the suffragette movement and the anti-apartheid campaign as examples. Maybe I/we can take some inspiration from this.

Once this was completed we ventured out into the sunshine and enjoyed an afternoon sitting in a boat on Lake Geneva, zigzagging across and taking in the sights.

23rd August – London

Because Sabrina is yet to take up the post of engagement and participation officer for London and to allow her to familiarise herself with the training package for service user involvement, the workshop that was planned before Elizabeth resigned was delivered today by Claire Garley and myself at the Corman Campus in London. I was supported today by Nicki, who is about to take the role of DEEP/KMPT volunteer coordinator for our local region. It was great to do this day with Nicki, to give her the opportunity of seeing service user involvement, which will be part of her role, albeit today with the Alzheimer's Society. It also gave Nicki and me a good opportunity to get to know each other and to talk about the Forget Me Nots and the role that I helped facilitate and secure funding for, alongside Reinhard and Elizabeth. It's been frustrating not having someone in post any quicker but I'm delighted that we've now found someone with the quality of Nicki. After the service user training workshop, Nicki accompanied me in going across to meet Andrew James for the first time in a café close to where the workshop was being held, to begin to move forward the new book project.

29th August – London

With Reinhard's support I was able as always to engage in discussions at today's DAA steering group meeting. A packed agenda included updates on the Seldom Heard Groups call to action, planning for the annual conference which again I am very happy to be invited to contribute towards, and an update from Kelly Kaye who, as the DAA Partnership Manager, led on the crucial hospitals project. After the steering group meeting, it was a mixture of emotions because it was sad to see the departure of Phil Freeman, who for the last couple of years has been leading the DAA and who has brought a great deal of commitment and energy to the role. I've enjoyed working with Phil, but now the time is right for him to move on and work with a different organisation. I was able to go for a while with Reinhard to Phil's leaving event at the Habit, located close to the Crutched Friars offices.

30th August – London

The Alzheimer's Society Grants Advisory Panel (GAP) meeting, at Crutched Friars, supported by Michael Blackburn, who is continuing to be able to provide support to people like myself through his employment on the KMPT bank.

2nd September – Canterbury

The Canterbury Pilgrims SURP group joined together today to walk as part of the Kent Memory Walk to raise funds for the Alzheimer's Society. The walk began at the University of Kent with approximately 1500 walkers in attendance. I was honoured to be asked to say some opening words from the stage, to thank people for supporting the event and to say a little about my views on the importance of the Alzheimer's Society, and how today's walk will help their work. Following this, I was invited to start the walk by cutting the ribbon.

Speaking of walks, yesterday I strolled along to pick some blackberries which the late summer sun is swelling and ripening. At one time I made a lot of juice; I do this less now, but maybe this fresh and freely available fruit along with some apples from a wayside tree will encourage me.

7th September – London

A very packed day in London with Rosemary, beginning in Whitehall with a meeting at the Department of Health, where we discussed around the table a way of following up and utilising the Dementia Statements. Subsequent to that, we had lunch 'on the hoof', making our way over to Waterloo for the next Young Onset Dementia workstream meeting.

When I got home that evening, in the post was a copy of the Alzheimer's Society Christmas catalogue. Featured in the opening was a message from myself and a rather prominent illustration of the *Walk the Walk, Talk the Talk* book, which was available within the catalogue.

11th September – Canterbury

People think that I am well organised and never late or miss a meeting; well today is an example of how I'm not always clear on what I'm doing. Rosemary and I arrived a week early for a talk connected to the U3A garden club that we belong to. We'd got the dates wrong – it should be next week and not this week, so I'm not always as organised as perhaps people think.

12th September – London
Following on from a recent research GAP meeting, today Nicki was able to join me again, this time for a board meeting for the Alzheimer's Society Research Network held at the Arbor City Hotel. Afterwards, it was lovely to be able to introduce Nicki to Lisa and Jess in order to have a catch-up with those two lovely people.

15th September – Canterbury
The annual talk to Year 3 occupational therapy students at Canterbury Christ Church University which as always I really enjoy as it reconnects me to the role of teacher.

16th September – Canterbury
For some time I have struggled to cope with dealing with shops, particularly large shops such as supermarkets and department stores, so I was quite determined to take myself along to Morrisons to pick up some bits and pieces that Rosemary and I required. I found it really hard and I couldn't get out of the shop quickly enough.

18th September – Canterbury
Rosie Duffield, Canterbury's newly elected Labour MP, was able to join the SURP meeting today and listen to our thoughts and concerns about dementia. Clearly Rosie has a sense of compassion towards people and some knowledge of dementia through family members, which certainly helped the conversation and our engagement with her. We look forward to hopefully collaborating in future.

19th September – London
DAA quarterly meeting with Reinhard, which saw the launch of the Seldom Heard Groups call to action and then on to an IDEAL programme advisory group meeting in the afternoon. Rosemary and I attended the

DAA in the morning with Reinhard, and left at lunchtime in order to fulfil the obligation for IDEAL. We then reconvened with friends, including Reinhard and Toby, afterwards. Rachael Litherland came with us, and Nada joined us later.

22nd September – Canterbury

I'm always delighted to meet with a new year's cohort of students, and today's group of eight look a very promising bunch. I enjoyed the hour I spent with them alongside Chris Norris. Over the past six years many lovely young people have come into my world through this placement programme and have given me genuine person-centred support, alongside which I hope I have contributed positively to their experience. Intergenerational working has enormous potential for all involved and I hope that others look at what we do in this area and seek to build upon it.

25th September – Canterbury

Alongside *Keith Oliver's Story* on YouTube, occasionally I look at the BBC film that utilises the footage made for the first *Victoria Derbyshire* programme on the subject of dementia back in 2015, which covered my, Wendy's and Christopher's story. I noticed today that that particular film has now surpassed 50,000 views in about two years. This prompted me to contact Jim Reed, the reporter who made the initial film, and ask him to consider if there is any possibility of revisiting the story now that it's two years old, and making a follow-up with Wendy, Christopher and myself. I wonder how he and the BBC will feel about this.

Alongside watching wildlife programmes which seem to dominate our choice of TV viewing these days, we are blessed to have nightly visits by up to three hedgehogs who we enjoy watching eat cat food which we place on our patio for them. We hope that eating this meal each day will help see them through their winter hibernation.

26th September – Canterbury

Reinhard came to my house today to work with me on an article to be published in the FPOP newsletter. This will focus on our friendship and collaboration following on from the talk we did at this year's FPOP conference. Our idea is to show the coming together of minds and experience from a common perspective but different objective. I'm really pleased and energised from the opportunity to do this and sense its importance in providing professionals and service users with a model to draw from. Indeed, this is a continuation of the concept we began with Ian Asquith back in 2011–2012 which culminated with our ADI poster presentation.

27th September – London

Full steering group meeting of the Young Onset Dementia Network near Kings Cross. During an informative presentation by Peter Watson, Rosemary's mind wandered for a moment when Peter was talking about RCTs – randomised controlled trials. Her experience of RCTs was very different based upon her work as a dental nurse where it meant root canal treatment! Both useful and maybe at times painful for those involved!

Great to see Donna, the new National Development Manager, really embracing the role.

28th September – Canterbury

After months of planning today we were able to unveil the first session of the Dreams and Visions writing project. This is the first of ten planned over the next few weeks using the Learning Lab within Beaney Library in Canterbury as our venue and base. Liz, joint project director with myself, outlined the aims of the project and fired everyone with enthusiasm for the task ahead. No one has attempted this before – to write a short film – and we all left feeling inspired.

When I got home after the writing session I felt excited and energised by the activities and went straight into an international Dementia Friends presentation being conducted as an Alzheimer's Society-led webinar involving eight people from around the world. The intention of this piece of work was to draw together professional organisations who are seeking to develop the Dementia Friends initiative in their own country, and the Alzheimer's Society asked me to express my views based upon my experience.

Then in the evening, Rosemary and I watched John Bishop interviewing David Walliams. I really like both men as comedians and as human beings. John Bishop's chat show really opens up the celebrity and draws deeply into their personality and past, but alongside this there is always humour. I liken the conversations in these programmes to the compassion-focused therapy sessions that I'm currently participating in with Yvette. One interesting aside is that David Walliams talks about his book *Camp David* which I have no recall of either owning or reading, but it's sitting on my bookshelf in front of me as I write my diary now.

29th September – London

Despite the mixed experience of helping with the judging at the National Dementia Awards last year, Rosemary and I were encouraged to again take part this year. Today we travelled to the Metropolitan Hotel to judge the category of inspirational leaders of care homes. This was a much better experience than last year for both of us, due in part to it being a different category and also to the fact that the co-judge was Emma Hewat, who was very easy to work with. She's also seen my film on YouTube and therefore knew me from that. Some of the nominees were really good, and it was a very close-run thing between them. However, we did manage to arrive at a unanimous decision between Emma, Rosemary and myself which we were all very happy about.

1st October – Canterbury

I hesitate from saying that I don't dream because I know that people do dream but don't always recall them. This is the case for me because I can honestly say that I don't remember dreams. Last night, or rather this morning, was an exception. I woke at 6 a.m. in the middle of a very bad dream. The dream involved living in the middle of a civil war and not knowing who was friend and who was foe. It was immensely distressing. Alongside that, someone very close to me said at the end of the dream that I am 'all talk', to which I responded, 'That's all I've got left.'

It wasn't a good night because Rosemary, struggling to sleep and consequently going downstairs at 2.20 a.m., missed the last two stairs and fell to the ground; although very badly shaken, she was very fortunate not to have seriously hurt herself.

8th October – Canterbury

The value of good friends who I've known for a long time and the value of remaining connected to others from one's past was illustrated today when I was visited by friends from our student days, Dave and Sarah Kerry and Anne and Tats, who spent most of the day with us at our house. Friends to me are increasingly important, and to have longstanding ones from our student days is a real bonus, and illustrates and reinforces the importance I attach to loyalty, both given and received. Today reminded me of a quote by Franz Kafka who wrote, 'Anyone who keeps the ability to see beauty never grows old.' I would add to this that the curious and interested also never grow old.

9th October – London
Three Nations Dementia Working Group meeting at the Crutched Friars with Rosemary, led by Adele Doherty now that Matt Murray has returned to his substantive post in managing the Research Network. Three important elements of the day were for me the presentation and dialogue with Maria McDonagh about the continued role of ambassadors within the society which, being one, I see as important; an advancement of our project to move forward the rights of people affected by dementia; and detailed discussion around the job description for the project officer post connected to the group, with an aim to have the person in post by 1st January. Afterwards Rosemary and I had a lovely catch-up with Rachel Hutchings and Katie Bennett at the society.

11th October – Canterbury
The OT project at Canterbury Christ Church University is now about halfway through and Pat Chung is reporting back to the small group her findings from interviews with couples who are accessing the Kent Enablement Service. It was great to have Abi's support again with this project.

13th October – Canterbury
Third nightmare in ten weeks, so something is happening to me during my sleep, although I don't know what. This time I felt bullied and scared because people were firing words at me. I woke distressed at 4 a.m. Rosemary had woken me previously as I was restless and also disturbing her sleep. I got up and read for a while and then went back to sleep.

16th October – Canterbury
A three-way teleconference between Philly, Rachel Hutchings, Rosemary and myself worked very well in preparation for a confidential meeting to be held with senior civil servants from the Department of Work and Pensions

and the Office of Disability Issues (ODI) regarding dementia, disability and rights. Our aim in this is to build upon my presentation to the United Nations and the consequent shortcomings of the government response.

17th October – Bromley and London

Through Angela, the chair of the Bromley Dementia Action Alliance, I was asked to speak at their launch today in Bromley, which I did supported by Nicki. I was also able to have a platform to promote *Walk the Walk, Talk the Talk* which proved popular. Following this we met with Andrew James and signed the contract for the new book at the Jessica Kingsley offices in Collier Street.

18th October – London

Through the Alzheimer's Society Dementia Friendly Communities team, Liz Jennings, Rosemary and I were invited to the launch of the dementia-friendly cinemas initiative at a cinema in Hackney, London. It was a lovely event and the three of us listened to a series of interesting presentations, one of which was by a fellow ambassador from Kent, Lorraine Brown. Lorraine took to the podium and talked about her current frequent visits to the cinema, and her desire to continue to engage in watching good-quality modern films.

Liz and I were able to support this with comments we made to the audience which to a point challenged some aspects of other presentations, which appeared to focus solely on showing people with dementia old films. There are many old films which we all enjoy re-watching, but it is a shame to exclude people with dementia from the opportunity to enjoy more modern films, especially those which are well made and brilliantly acted.

Travelling back on the high-speed train with Liz and Rosemary, there was an interesting aside where the guard, making an announcement on the train, spoke in a slow tone of voice I aim to utilise as one of the characters – a barista – in my film script for the Dreams and Visions project.

19th October – Canterbury

After the third Dreams and Visions project session today I met April Doyle and Liz to discuss my next book, followed in the afternoon by a writing session with Reinhard to prepare for a presentation we are due to make in

Newquay next month. We have been invited to outline what Kent are doing in connection with co-production and psychology for older adults, and how this may help encourage the commissioners in Cornwall to provide greater resources in that county. The meeting with Liz and April involved sharing ideas around proof-reading, general ideas for the book (including a title), and how the use of a Dictaphone could work.

20th October – London

Continuing our involvement in the Angela Project through a PPI meeting at Dementia UK headquarters with Rosemary, and then afterwards in the same building we held a meeting in the basement with Deborah and Edward, who are senior civil servants from the Department of Disability Issues. This followed up the telephone planning meeting that Rachel, Philly and I had a few days ago. The purpose of this meeting was to share with the senior civil servants our experiences of dementia, something along the lines of what Philly and I covered with the UN, and to give them an opportunity to be able to speak on behalf of the government, because no one seems particularly happy with their response to the UN. Beyond this I hope this will support the move forward and seek ways of achieving easy gains for the benefit of people with dementia alongside long-term aspirations.

23rd October – Canterbury

Nada visited me today from London to discuss a chapter in a book that she's writing with the support of folk like myself on the use of technology in supporting people with dementia. I explained my views on technology being a useful tool, but nothing more than that. She was also able to meet Karon and William, who are staying with us at the moment, which was very nice. Following this I went to Gregory House to see Yvette for the final session of therapy. But I went three days too early! Again a case of me not being as well organised as I would wish. In the evening we had a lovely family party at Cote Brasserie for James's 35th birthday. It's scary how the years have flown by.

24th October – London

Chris Norris, Carol Fordyce and myself, supported by Andrew Coleman, one of this year's students, attended a SURP review meeting at Crutched Friars, led by Lesley, the engagement and participation officer for the Midlands. We looked at ways in which the SURPs can be energised through discussing how they currently function and how they might continue in the future. We also shared ideas around a name change as apparently the acronym SURP isn't viewed positively by everybody.

Representatives at the meeting came from three SURPs – Canterbury, Ilkeston and one in London. After the meeting I saw Katie Bennett and Matt Murray at Crutched Friars for a catch-up chat.

26th October – Canterbury

After this morning's Dreams and Visions workshop, it was in fact the final therapy session with Yvette today. I was able to go through the workshop with Yvette and explained that whilst sometimes being comfortable in a leadership role, often I do wish to slip into the background where the pressure and expectations of others (and myself) are rather less. We also talked about the way I was structuring the support of the students for the writers by keeping the partnerships loose, fluid and dynamic so that each person had a different partner for each session, thus keeping it fresh without anyone feeling too attached to an individual.

27th October – Canterbury

Attended a Forget Me Nots buddies meeting led by psychologist Jo Vidal, alongside Chris, Carol, Melvyn, Carolina and Mark, with Andrew Coleman supporting. The idea is that we would give some peer support to people who have just been diagnosed in our locality. This could work well if it's structured correctly and supported adequately, and the idea takes me back to some meetings we had five years ago with the SILK team at Thanington Resource Centre, which coincided with the Memorabilia group setting up the Maidstone mentors.

30th October – Canterbury

Reinhard came to visit me at home today for the second writing session to prepare our presentation for the conference in Cornwall. We also discussed travel plans for the three of us, which will involve travelling from Canterbury to St Pancras, across to Paddington, down to Par in Cornwall and then changing to another train to Newquay. Quite a trek, but it will be exciting. The psychologist in Cornwall, Rebecca Reed, has been incredibly good at communicating with Reinhard and me in the preparation for this event and is keen that we travel and speak to support her efforts to get more resources for psychology allocated to support older adults in the county.

2nd November – London

Alzheimer's Society Research Network South East conference at Crutched Friars supported by Darshi, which drew together members of the network to hear two keynote speakers, one talking about the value of cognitive behavioural therapy and one outlining some important drug trials, so both portfolios and aspects of the Research Network were well represented and delivered. There was then a round-table discussion focusing on how the network can move forward. My key point was around increasing the membership of people with dementia in the network and seeking ways of better enabling participation of people with dementia in research projects at the outset, rather than just when the project is up and running.

3rd November – Canterbury

Whether it is by chance, by coincidence, or something lodged in my subconscious after yesterday, today I had a telephone call from Simon Evans, a senior researcher at Worcester University, regarding the idea of a research project that both he and I can submit to the Alzheimer's Society for potential funding, which seeks to focus on the impact that dementia has on men. This idea began with a conversation that Simon and I had a while ago at a VERDe meeting in London. A potentially interesting new project for me to be involved in.

In the year since *Walk the Walk, Talk the Talk* was published, it has exceeded my hopes and expectations by selling over 500 copies, which has raised about £2500 for the Alzheimer's Society and Innovations in Dementia. I will promote it for another year to 18 months in the hope that this figure can be doubled and therefore match the performance of *Welcome to Our World*. Both books feature in the Alzheimer's Society online shop, with *Walk the Walk, Talk the Talk* also having a prominent position in their catalogue.

6th–8th November – Exeter

Rosemary and I travelled to Exeter to allow me to speak about the IDEAL project at an event called the Economic and Social Research Festival of Social Science. Today started with catching up with Steve Milton for a coffee alongside browsing the shops, museum and cathedral to get a sense of what Exeter has to offer. This was followed by a lovely meal and conversation with Ruth Lamont, one of the project researchers, who we have met before. She then took us to the venue in good time for me to prepare for my talk.

I was very pleased to be able to speak on stage alongside Catherine Quinn and Alex Hillman from the IDEAL project. Professor Linda Clare and Ruth were in the audience for the talk and, as always, at times during the talk I was grateful to be able to focus upon friendly and familiar faces to give me extra confidence.

9th November – Canterbury

Our Dreams and Visions project is going very well and today was workshop six of ten, after which I met Alan to discuss the Canterbury Sound, a style of music that emerged from Canterbury in the late 1960s and early 1970s. Alan was put in touch with me because he is studying a master's and writing a thesis on the Canterbury Sound. Liz thought he would be someone who I could usefully engage and talk with to our mutual benefit, and through this I could find out more about the background to the story that I'm using in my film script.

10th November – Canterbury

Today was the monthly Forget Me Nots meeting and a chance to celebrate the group's fifth birthday. The party atmosphere lightened what has at times become a 'coliseum' type of environment where some members express personal and at times vitriolic comments at other members of the group.

14th November – London and Manchester

I have been invited to a meeting at the Department of Health building in Whitehall, entitled the Experience and Satisfaction Measures Task and Finish Group. Following this, with sandwiches in our bags, Rosemary and I dashed up to Manchester for the 3 Nations Dementia Working Group meeting at the Alzheimer's Society managers' conference. We arrived in time to meet with other members of the Department of Health, who wanted to get the views of our group on a range of issues. Then in the evening we attended the Alzheimer's Society dinner, during which there was an opportunity to celebrate the work of individuals. I was able to speak on behalf of service users, thanking everyone who worked for the Alzheimer's

Society by extolling the amazing folk who work so hard at grass-roots level. Also, whilst not making any apology, I got the microphone for a second time and expressed gratitude to Jeremy Hughes for his caring leadership of the society, without whom many worthwhile initiatives would remain on the drawing board.

15th November – Manchester

Day two of the conference involving 3 Nations Dementia Working Group discussions about projects that we wish to proceed with. We had five projects to discuss and decide upon. The group unanimously decided to support initially the one that I proposed and talked about, which focused around human rights.

16th November – Canterbury

After an informative walk and a conversation focusing on the Canterbury Sound with Alan, it was then into the Beaney for another writing workshop to continue to work on the scripts which the eight of us are currently seeking to produce. I left promptly at 12 noon and met Rosemary to travel to London for the Young Onset Dementia workstream meeting, where again our main focus was the GP guide. The group had kindly delayed the start to allow Rosemary and me the time to attend.

17th November – Canterbury

Today was a care programme approach meeting at St Martin's with Richard Brown and Yvette, to see how I am and to look forward with my care plan now that therapy has come to an end. It was agreed that I would see Richard in mid-February before going on holiday to Australia. I know how fortunate I have been to receive this level of support from Yvette, and whilst I am concerned that it is coming to an end I recognise the continuation of Richard's support alongside placing the responsibility upon me to utilise some of the strategies introduced to me by Yvette over recent months. After this I went to a DEEP, BPS and Forget Me Nots meeting in Thanington to discuss methods and ideas the BPS can employ to better support people with dementia.

21st–24th November – Cornwall

After in-depth planning between Reinhard and me, supported by Rebecca Reed, we are now in Cornwall with the opportunity to speak at a staff conference for Cornwall Partnership NHS Foundation Trust, organised by Rebecca, the sole older adults psychologist in the county. Reinhard and I spoke about our work together and the need to invest further in Cornwall in order to meet their growing demand. Rosemary and I had extra days in the area as tourists, which we utilised by shopping in Truro and going for a beach walk near the hotel situated in Porth. We had a lovely time, although it was extremely blustery with gales blowing in off the Atlantic.

27th November and 2nd December – Canterbury

Two more writing sessions at my house with Reinhard. This time we'd been asked to contribute a commentary to a new version of Tom Kitwood's book *Dementia Reconsidered*. This new book is being edited by Professor Dawn Brooker because it's now 20 years since this seminal book was published. Dawn invited Reinhard and me to read and provide an updated commentary on Chapter 5, entitled 'The Experience of Dementia', which we feel honoured and privileged to do. We began today by reading the original text and scribbling down our shared and separate experiences and ideas on the original work and how the experience of dementia is different 20 years after Kitwood's writing. Next week we will meet again and complete the piece before sending it off to Dawn.

28th November – Canterbury

Despite the late start to the monthly face-to-face sessions with the two students supporting me this year, Darshi, Andrew and I met today for what was a really good session. Our main focus was on getting to know each other and talking about plans for the forthcoming year. They are clearly two enthusiastic young people, and I gave them the task for next time of preparing an interview with me for my new book, which can then be included in the book.

30th November – London

DAA steering group meeting at Crutched Friars with Reinhard. Now Phil Freeman has left, Kelly Kaye has taken over and this period is seeing her starting to establish herself following this step-up. The agenda was a mix of reports from ongoing work and final plans for the annual conference which is in a week's time.

6th December – London

DAA annual conference in London with Rosemary and Reinhard, followed by a debriefing after the meeting at the local hostelry. I really enjoy these days – such an excellent blend of listening to interesting speakers, networking and, if given the opportunity, a chance to express myself on a topic which is important to me (in this case the rights of those affected by dementia). As Nigel Hullah is unwell I was asked to read the talk Nigel had diligently prepared, and I hope I did justice to his powerful words.

7th December – Canterbury

Tenth and final screenwriting session for the Dreams and Visions project. Everyone – writers and supporters alike – came away feeling immensely proud of our achievements but also a little sad to see the sessions come to an end. Of the ten people with dementia who started the project, seven have stayed the course, which, given the challenge placed in front of people to come so often and to write in a genre no one would have even considered a few months ago, is quite amazing. The range and quality of the scripts is astonishing. Now the challenge is to lift them from paper into action. To do this in the new year we will liaise with the Marlowe Theatre for a public showing using a rehearsed reading format whilst we seek funding to make the scripts into short films.

8th December – Canterbury

After the Forget Me Nots meeting I rang Melvyn to check how he is, as I've done every four to five days or so following the very sad and sudden death of his dear wife Jan recently. As a friend I am concerned about how he is coping and talk to him about how he's eating, if he's shopping and getting food in, if he is getting out and seeing his family. I usually close by checking if he is coming to the next Forget Me Nots meeting.

10th December – London

An early snowfall didn't stop us travelling to London and exploring the area around Spitalfields Market prior to being involved on an interview panel tomorrow with the Alzheimer's Society. Overnight we stayed at the Grange City Hotel in London and met with Mycal Miller to discuss my film, which also enabled the three of us to touch base about how we're keeping. He gave me a DVD entitled *I Bought a Vampire Motorcycle*, a film he'd made some years ago starring Neil Morrissey. He knows it's not 'my cup of tea' but I do plan to try and watch it, maybe after Christmas.

11th December – London

Helping with interviews for a director post at the Alzheimer's Society with Rosemary and Hilary Doxford, supported by Claire Garley and Cris, a member of Alzheimer's Society staff. We hope Sally Copley will be the successful candidate. Her Skype interview very much reminded me of an interview with Lisa Bogue three and a half years ago. Similar but very different.

13th December – London

A 3 Nations Dementia Working Group meeting at the Hotel Indigo in London to discuss and decide upon a logo for the group. Participating today were Wendy Mitchell, Chris and Jayne Roberts, Rosemary and myself, supported by Kim and Vivienne from the Alzheimer's Society. In the afternoon, Rosemary and I went over to Kings Cross to participate in our six-monthly Young Dementia Network meeting with Chris and Jayne.

15th December – Canterbury

Liz Jennings visited me today to discuss closing phase one and moving forward to phase two of the Dreams and Visions project. In the afternoon, out of loyalty to Janet Lloyd, I attended her leaving do at St Martin's Hospital.

Jim Reed emailed from the BBC regarding wanting to do some filming next week, but with Christmas so close, I said there's no way I could do that – it has to be done after Christmas.

18th December – Canterbury

Jan Brooks's funeral and wake at Melvyn's daughter Victoria's house. There was a very large turnout, including a number of people from the Forget Me Nots group, to pay our respects and to support our friend Melvyn.

One early consequence of having dementia was around issues with my balance, and regularly since then I have tried to do balancing exercises. Initially I was only managing less than ten seconds on either leg. Now, by regularly doing balancing exercises, currently I am able to maintain my balance for 170 seconds on my right leg and approximately 180 seconds on my left leg, which obviously is a substantial improvement. Also, previously, because of difficulties with my balance, I would often use a stick when out walking; now I seldom require it but do still occasionally carry it with me folded in my bag. In addition to that, in order to try and improve my cardiovascular circulation, I do regular exercises using an ab-rocker.

19th December – Canterbury

The second monthly meeting at my house with Andrew and Darshi, the placement students. Today we followed up the homework task that I set them where I asked them to write an interview and then conduct the interview with me about the book. We recorded it in writing and then they typed up my responses. In addition, they gave me support with some IT issues and typing the first Dear Alzheimer's letter for the new book.

20th December – Canterbury

Approximately every four weeks I continue to meet with Eric and Jen at Nero's. Having completed the study of the Gospel According to John, we're moving on to the Gospel According to Luke. Although not able to attend Eric's church, I do listen to services on a podcast, complete the homework he sets, reflect upon lessons we discuss as a threesome, and enjoy the friendship we share at these meetings.

25th December – Reculver

Ever since spending Christmas 1989 on a sun-drenched Australian beach we have as a family packed a picnic hamper on Christmas Day and headed off to a Kent beach to either soak up some winter sun or dodge the icy rain. Irrespective of the weather it's champagne and 'cheesy footballs' on the beach or in a nearby seafront shelter! There are so many places to visit and we enjoy the challenge of trying to find somewhere new nearby; this year we made our way to set up camp on the beach in the shadows of the Saxon church and Roman fort at Reculver, near Herne Bay.

30th December – Canterbury

Once the family had left us after the Christmas break, I spent the rest of the year recovering and sorting my office, as I did last year. This enabled me to bring the old year to a close and get ready for 2018. I also took the opportunity to check the films on YouTube, which showed me 33,500 views for *Keith Oliver's Story* (I jokingly tell audiences I am only responsible for 25,000 of these), running now at about 200 views a week, and 56,000 for the BBC film, with about 450 views per week. I must tell Jim Reed at the BBC this before his visit in a few days to film an update with me.

31st December – Canterbury

Whether or not it was because I have been thinking about today being the seventh anniversary of being given the diagnosis of dementia, last night I had a very strange dream again. This time there was no civil war, or shouting aggressive people from my life; in fact it was quite a sedate dream but nonetheless quite disturbing.

In the dream I was on a train travelling back from London, something I do now quite often, and was reflecting upon my current busy life and the activities I am involved in as an ambassador, activist, envoy, husband, dad, granddad, friend and person. Reinhard's words expressed to me five years ago about professionals wanting a slice of my time have proved so prophetic. I get a sense of achievement, which boosts my vulnerable self-esteem, from helping others and from being wanted, which in turn makes me feel respected and valued. I worried in my dream about what I would do if I let anyone down and when I can no longer continue to engage in these meaningful activities. I know at some point the current door which is open will close. Sometimes, and this was the case in the dream, I wonder who I am; how am I defined by myself, and by others – who is the real ME in deMEntia? I am the person behind the occasionally worn mask of wellness when the dementia makes more mischief than I can easily hide.

As I often do, to seek reassurance I turned to music in my dream, and during lulls in conversation with my faceless companion I had music 'worming' in my mind – a Paul Simon favourite, surprisingly not, given the situation, 'Homeward Bound', but the extra verse from 'The Boxer' about years rolling by me and changes upon changes but we are more or less the same; 'While I Am Here', which I see as my signature tune and use frequently to support my talks; and 'Won't Give In', which when I am low gives me great strength. The journey on the train takes about 55 minutes; I cannot say how long the dream took to unfold. The journey with dementia has to date taken seven and a half years. Sometimes when I look back it seems a long, long way from there to here and I wonder how much longer I am to carry on travelling.

Time will tell, but sunset is often the most memorable time of the day.

Sometime in 2017

Dear Alzheimer's

As I sit down and seek to pen this final letter I want to remind you that all these words written in my letters and diary are my own, not co-written or thoughts shared with a ghost writer. Although often hard for me to convey my thoughts in words – spoken and written – for me no one else could accurately capture my thoughts and words. You might think at times I would slink away and lick the wounds generated by feeling sorry for myself; this, 'dear Alzheimer's', as you are realising through these letters, and from residing inside my head and life, is simply not my style.

One of my main attempts to live well with you is to focus upon living in the day, but also planning one or two positive things for the near future, and then going out and doing my very best to ensure that they happen. Often this is despite your attempts to undermine both my planning and then my ability to bring this about.

I know that you, depression and Screwtape, C.S. Lewis's apprentice nephew of the devil, lurk together as a terrible triad of fog and mayhem, and I hope that after you have read my final letter you and your dark allies will slip back to your murky depths. I am energised and take inspiration from those who genuinely care. I see in these people's eyes and feel in their heart not sympathy but empathy, encouragement and their generous sense of positive compassion. One key strategy I use, and will utilise, to change your long-held views is that *every* negative comment requires four positive ones to redress the balance and restore those who show sincerity and love. The truth about life and faith sits centrally in all of this.

I also know that you cannot resist peering over my shoulder as I write and you seek to undermine my efforts. So you will have seen how many gains against you there have been since you came to reside inside my head. Amongst these gains are improved diagnosis rates; the combined efforts of the Dementia Action Alliance; communities uniting against you as dementia-friendly communities which effectively engage with all sectors and age groups; the Young Dementia Network, which has galvanised groups of professionals and service users for the benefit of younger people with dementia in a way that was unthinkable back in 2010; and the amazing efforts of so many people allied to DEEP, which weaves a positive route through my diary. But, 'dear Alzheimer's', you and I know this progress is in many ways fragile and inconsistent across our country. I can still sincerely say that I hope tomorrow is better than today for those living with you.

Happy endings to stories or those concluding with 'and they lived happily ever after' do not usually happen with you as the central character. Having said that, when our relationship began back in 2010, if someone had said to me that in 2017 I would be doing this, and suggested what I would achieve in the years between, I would certainly have grabbed the offer with both hands. You tell me you are a servant of death, and at some point your master will take me, but it is not in your power to decide when that will be. There is a far more powerful, positive force which will determine that, as shown in my growing faith. As the lights start to dim I do intend to leave the 'party' before the last waltz.

It has been a long way from there to here, but hopefully, 'dear Alzheimer's', there is still a long way to go. Hear my words, read my words, 'dear Alzheimer's', I will finish writing before you stop reading them. Until which I intend to stay a while longer in the sun.

With frosty regards

Keith

Closing words

I was recently at Canterbury West station with Rosemary waiting for a train to London for a dementia meeting. I bumped into a former head teacher colleague who I hadn't seen since my retirement. The look on his face suggested that he had seen a ghost. His opening words were, 'Hello Keith, I thought you were dead.'

We then proceeded to chat about what I was currently doing and I reinforced the point that I was still very much alive. Thoughts of Mark Twain came to mind with the quote 'The report of my death was greatly exaggerated.'

This conversation both shocked and surprised me. Maybe it shouldn't have done, because what he thought was 'How could this person still be alive eight years after disclosing he had Alzheimer's?', and then 'How could a person with Alzheimer's look, speak and act in the way they are doing?' There is a growing number of people living with dementia who are actively raising awareness around the true picture of the condition, but clearly there's still some way to go.

Since he thought I was no longer in the land of the living, I decided to post a message on Facebook, alongside a photograph of me taken that day by Rosemary. The response from friends was unsurprisingly supportive, as they knew there was still a bit of life in this old boy. This, alongside an enormous groundswell of love and positivity generated from the Canterbury Residents Group, was both humbling and moving. Those who responded clearly do understand.

The end of a year is a time to take stock and, as the ancient Roman god Janus did, to look back at the old year and forward to the new one.

Another highlight I thought would not happen is that new friends – many of them falling into the label of 'professional friends' as coined by Reinhard and myself – have entered into my world and so enriched it. I am now a real hoarder of *everything* as I try to cling to the flotsam and jetsam of life, and memory and friends sometimes fall into this net. So to have new people coming into my life who add to the richness of my experience is so encouraging. I have been treated as part of the 'family' by those working at the Alzheimer's Society and Young Dementia UK, who are real heroes not just for me but for the many others they serve, support and befriend in the true sense of the word.

There are many more highlights, but those who have shared them with me know what they are without me falling into any traps that can await one writing this kind of piece.

I will keep going with these roles for a bit longer despite the trials and tribulations that dementia throws my way. I think about giving up at times and even wonder what the point is. I doubt myself daily, and in turn I am horrified to admit I doubt others who deserve better from me. But then other days, the sun does shine, and by this light I see life more clearly and the fog recedes.

I mentioned Janus earlier, and I close with another story from ancient times which I was always identified with at Blean – Pandora's Box. I trust that the main message of this legend of *hope* comes through in this writing and I hope that you all are able to live well despite what challenges life presents to you.

Along with hope, the other most important word to me in the English language is *love*, and by sharing that with you, the reader, I close.

Film script

RECONCILIATION (AN OUTLINE)
FILM SCRIPT BY KEITH OLIVER

Scene 1: SOMEONE being filmed in washed-out tones
(*almost black and white*)

Rick Shoreham, aged about 70, on his own in a room with music on in the background.

Music is 'Winter Wine' – instrumental intro and first few lyrics of a Caravan track (approx 45 seconds).

In the corner of the room are some CDs, books, etc., and a guitar propped up on a stand, maybe an amp also. The guy is listening and seeming to be in a daze. No sound other than the music.

The daze is disturbed by his daughter coming into the room.

WANTS SOMETHING

Conversation take place along the lines of 'Come on, Dad, what are you doing today?', 'Nothing much', etc. She is calm and encouraging, he is defensive and knocking back her help – not aggressively but almost defeated/depressed in his manner.

His hands are a little shaky and his voice uncertain.

She tells him what his doctor has said about being busy, keeping engaged, active, etc. to ward off his dementia, which is just beginning to influence his life. He is dismissive of this – can't do this/that, haven't got a problem, etc. He is in denial.

She tries to encourage him to play his guitar as he was listening to the music of his former band on CD.

He tries and is frustrated. Stops and gently puts it down – 'Won't do this again, Rosie,' he says. 'I want to remember how it was, and not feel how it is now. I'm told to reminisce, so that's what I'm doing.'

Scene 2: AND TAKES ACTION

Rosie on her own watching YouTube film of her dad's old Canterbury Sound group The Stourmen (aka Caravan circa late 1960s, etc.).

Music – Winter Wine (by Caravan) at about 2 min 50 secs for a minute or so.

She is also flicking through old photos of her dad from the days of the band.

Goes on computer – looks at Facebook for the names on the photos to see what she might find.

No dialogue, just the background music.

MEETS CONFLICT

Rick comes in – 'What are you doing with the photos and listening to that rubbish?'

Rosie for first time gets cross – 'You thought you were bulletproof/ armour-plated when you were drinking too much, smoking too much stuff and womanising in the band. It's no wonder that Mum left you when we were kids, and now you're leaving yourself, Dad.'

Rick goes over to her, silently, picks up the photos and looks at them. Music still on.

'Didn't know you were that good, Dad.'

'No, neither did I,' says Rick and leaves the room with Rosie still looking at her computer.

PROBLEM/OBSTACLES (*filming in gradual increase of colour tone*)

'How can I get them together, how can I bring Dad to see the benefits of meeting up with his old buddies and reconciling them?' – Rosie talking/thinking out loud/thought bubble/split screen filming her typing and sending a message.

Goes through Facebook – finds grown-up children of the three other band members – sends them messages – gets positive responses.

Scene 3: Same setting a week or so later – LEADING TO A CRISIS

Rosie is seen checking her messages and muttering to herself about the positive responses of the band members.

Scene 4: Rick's lounge

Rosie: 'Come on, smarten your ideas and yourself – we are going out for a coffee.'

They go to a café in Canterbury and Rosie tells Rick about her plan to go to the cathedral gate where there had been so many memories of the band days and where the band had started as buskers back in the late 1960s.

Scene 5: The café – LEADING TO A CLIMAX (speak to manager of Kudos restaurant to use for filming this scene)

Humour with slow-speaking and slow-thinking barista repeating the coffee order – 'cap-o chi-no, lar-tay'.

Rosie has the band photos with her and shows her dad. He seems a bit more positive towards them and his fingers begin to indicate playing chords very discreetly – no longer shaking. Seems a bit more relaxed. He's now talking and Rosie is listening.

He mentions the foolishness of the band falling out and 40 years spent not contacting each other and how that has played on his mind. Rosie says nothing but smiles and listens.

Scene 6: Outside St Thomas Church Hall

Walk from Kudos to the cathedral gate via St Thomas Church Hall. Rick stops Rosie and tells her how this also used to be a venue the band played back in the late 1960s.

Music score in background – 'In the Land of Grey and Pink' by Caravan (the instrumental section after about 3 mins).

Scene 7: Outside the cathedral gate in the Buttermarket – WHICH IS RESOLVED (*in colour by this scene*)

The other band members are there first – they have clearly kept in touch and still feel positive towards each other but Rick has been outside of this loop since the split 40 years previously.

Buskers are playing quietly and can be heard (shown on film?). Their volume gradually decreases as the banter and conversation of the band takes place.

Rosie leads her dad towards the group and then there is that sense of recognition. He looks at them and then at Rosie; she smiles back at her dad. No conversation. He walks towards the others and the group embrace, then banter ensues about gigs and how good/bad they were – 'Do you remember?'-type statements. Each has some photos that include Rick, and these now become a source of positive comments rather than the dismissive ones from earlier in the film.

Rosie backs out of the scene as this starts and leaves the old blokes to it.

History repeating itself – next to them the small group of young buskers who have been performing start an argument with each other about their music, blaming each other, etc., and the old guys look over, shake their heads and look at each other, and then walk away laughing with arms around each other's shoulders.

Soundtrack music playing in background – 'Golf Girl' by Caravan (the trumpet and guitar intro to the track – 30 seconds).

At the end play 'Love to Love You' by Caravan.

The End

RECONCILIATION
BY KEITH OLIVER

Scene 1: Rick's lounge

Music is playing: 'Winter Wine' by Caravan (from 45 seconds in). We see CDs, books, a guitar on a stand.

> RICK SHOREHAM *(70s) sits in the lounge listening to the music in a daze.*
>
> ROSIE – *Rick's daughter – enters the room. She is full of bustle in contrast to Rick's passive pose.*

ROSIE

Come on, Dad, what are you doing today?

Rick stirs, looks up at her, and mumbles sadly in response.

She stands, he is slouched.

She lays a hand on his shoulder. He remains statuesque.

CLOSE UP Rick's hands shaking. We hear Rick mutter an incomprehensible response.

CLOSE UP on Rosie.

ROSIE

Come on Dad, you know your doctor said it's good for you to keep busy.

Rick turns slightly away from her.

RICK

I don't want to do that.

ROSIE

You know it'll help you.

RICK

I haven't got a problem. Why do I need help?

ROSIE

Well, the doctor says that they think you've got dementia, Dad.

RICK

I haven't got dementia. My memory is good. I can remember my music. I can remember you. What more do I need?

Rosie walks to the guitar on the stand. As she walks, she speaks.

ROSIE

I've not seen you play your guitar in a while, Dad.

CLOSE UP on Rick's face. He looks thoughtful and uncertain.

CLOSE UP Rosie's hands passing Rick's guitar to him.

CLOSE UP Rick's shaking hands trying to play the strings and failing. Rick lays the guitar on the ground next to him.

RICK

I won't do this again, Rosie. I want to remember how it was, and not to feel how it is now.

ROSIE

But...

RICK

I'm told to reminisce, and that's what I'm doing, by listening to how we used to be.

Scene 2: Dining room in Rick's house

Music plays: 'Winter Wine' by Caravan, playing from 2 minutes 50 seconds in.

Rosie is watching a YouTube film of a 1960s group of four men performing music.

She flicks through an old photo album which lies on the table next to the computer.

It is pictures of her dad's band.

Rosie turns back to the computer. We see the screen as she goes onto Facebook.

She's typing in names, muttering to herself.

Rick enters, then hovers in the door opening as he sees the photo albums.

RICK

What are you doing with those photos, listening to that rubbish?

Rosie looks hurt and cross.

ROSIE

You thought you were bulletproof and armour-plated when you were drinking too much stuff and womanising in the band. It's no wonder Mum left when I was a kid, and now you're leaving yourself, Dad!

Rick goes silently over to Rosie.

He picks up and looks at some of the photos. He looks thoughtful.

Rosie is calming down as she watches her dad, and she joins him in looking at the photos.

ROSIE

Didn't know you were that good, Dad.

RICK

Neither did I.

Rick leaves the room.

Rosie turns back to the computer. She's typing on Facebook.

She gives up in exasperation and reaches for the phone.

CUT TO: Rosie stands by the window on the phone talking to a FRIEND.

ROSIE

Thing is, all I've got to go on is Facebook and some old photos. I mean, how do you reconcile people who haven't spoken in 40 years? ... Really? You can? That's great, thanks for all your help. I'll let you know how it goes. See you soon. Bye.

Rosie sits back at the computer, looking optimistic.

ROSIE

Right, tell me what to do...

Scene 3: Rick's dining room. WORDS ON SCREEN: One week later...

Rosie is checking her emails on the laptop, and muttering happily to herself.

She gets up and leaves the room.

Scene 4: Rick's lounge

The lounge is a mess.

Rick sits there, dishevelled, unshaven and slouching. He's clearly not taking care of himself.

ROSIE

Come on, Dad, smarten yourself up. We're going out for coffee.

Scene 5: Inside a café

Rosie and Rick sit at a table.

A waiter comes over. We see he has a badge reading 'Trainee Barista'.

ROSIE

I've had an idea, Dad.

WAITER *(speaking excessively slowly and boringly)*
Hello.

ROSIE

Hello. A cappuccino and a latte, please.

RICK *(chin on hand)*

I'm not sure what you've got in mind, Rosie.

WAITER *(hovering over Rick and Rosie – painfully slowly and tediously)*

Cappuccino...latte.

ROSIE

Yes, please.

She waits for the waiter to leave, but he stays.

She looks back at Rick, smiling, bemused but tolerant.

WAITER

Cappuccino...latte.

ROSIE

Thank you.

She turns to her father. She is making an effort to sound casual and jolly.

ROSIE

We're just going to go for a walk, Dad. You can tell me about some of the places where you played. You've not brought me to Canterbury since I was a kid.

RICK

I'm still not sure, Rosie. You're pushing me, and I'm not sure I want to be pushed.

WAITER *(who returns to the table looking puzzled)*

So that's a cappuccino and a latte?

ROSIE

Yes, please.

Rosie smiles at the waiter, who smiles in return before walking away.

ROSIE

I remember a place you used to tell me about – what was it? I think it was
an old hall – I can't remember any more than that, Dad.

RICK

That was St Thomas Church Hall. We had some good gigs there.

ROSIE

Wouldn't you like to show me?

*The waiter reappears, this time with a tray and two drinks which he offers
to Rosie and Rick.*

WAITER

Just to check, that was a cappuccino and a latte, right?

ROSIE *(kindly)*

That's right, thank you very much.

RICK

Mmm...

Rosie pulls out some loose photos she's brought with her.

*CUT TO: Close up – Rick's hands holding the photos. His hands are steady,
not shaking this time.*

CLOSE UP on Rick's face.

RICK

It's been 40 years, Rosie. Such a foolish argument. So stupid. 40 years
wasted. We've had no contact. You don't know, Rosie, how much that's
upset me over the years.

ROSIE

You should have said, Dad.

RICK

I've never spoken to anyone about it, Rosie. When you're in a band, it's like a family.

CLOSE UP on Rosie's face.

She smiles, listens and reaches for her now steady dad's hand.

Scene 6: Outside St Thomas Church Hall

Music plays: ' In the Land of Grey and Pink' by Caravan, starting at the 3-minute point.

Rick and Rosie are walking towards the hall from the High Street, past the Superdrug building.

Rick stops by the hall and holds Rosie's arm and they both look at the building, Rick looking deep in thought and Rosie smiling and looking at her dad.

RICK

This is the venue the band played back in '68

ROSIE

This is great, Dad. I am really enjoying today and I can't wait to hear more about your life in the band.

They walk on further hand in hand through the streets of Canterbury towards the cathedral.

Scene 7: The Buttermarket by the cathedral gate

Music continues from last scene (Caravan – 'In the Land of Grey and Pink').

Three men – GRAHAM, SID and PETE – stand together outside the cathedral gate.

They're laughing, clearly familiar with each other, joking and teasing each other.

Our view switches to a group of four young lads who are busking.

They play 'Love to Love You' by Caravan.

Rosie takes her dad's arm and leads him towards the group of three older men.

We see hesitant recognition appearing on Rick's face.

He's uncertain – he looks at them and looks back at Rosie.

Rosie gives a knowing smile.

The buskers' music fades.

Rick starts to walk towards the group, slightly more confident now.

The buskers' music starts up again.

Rick is smiling now – his first smile of the film.

The band see Rick and one by one they each hug him.

Then the three band members open out to receive Rick and the four embrace as one.

They begin to chat. We hear snatches of conversation.

GRAHAM
You've changed!

SID
Remember when...

PETE *(pulling out some photos from his pocket)*
I've brought these.

SID
I've got some too.

RICK
Oh – we've got some with us. Rosie – did you remember to bring the photos?

ROSIE
Here you go, Dad.

Rosie backs quietly away leaving her dad and the others happily talking together.

The young buskers begin to argue.

One of them has played an incorrect note or got the words wrong, or shown off.

We hear raised voices in disagreement which results in a heated argument between the young men.

Sid, Graham, Pete and Rick stop chatting and turn to watch the buskers.

The old guys are smiling knowing smiles, exchanging looks: they have been there, done that.

They each shake their heads.

They put their arms around each other's shoulders and walk off down Sun Street, chatting (inaudible).

Perhaps an upper body or whole body shot here.

Music cuts in – Caravan's original version of 'Love to Love You' which the Stourmen and the buskers 40 years apart each performed.

The End

Interview

Interview between Keith Oliver and Darshi and Andrew (support students from the University of Kent on placement with Kent and Medway Partnership Trust) about writing the book

To get to know you, can you describe yourself in two or three sentences?
I consider myself as an ex-teacher who now lives in Canterbury with dementia. Alongside this, I am married with three grown-up children and three rapidly growing-up grandchildren. I try to continue to enjoy a range of hobbies which alongside my dementia, ambassador and envoy roles keep me busy, and by being busy I am able to remain as well as possible.

What motivated you to write your first book?
I attended a writing course at Canterbury Christ Church University delivered by April Doyle which inspired me, and gave me the confidence to consider writing stories from my life in the hope that readers may be interested. This was then followed up with a further writing course designed for people with dementia delivered by Liz Jennings, which resulted in the unique and groundbreaking book *Welcome to Our World* back in 2014. This book was a collaborative project which I found very motivational, co-authored by eight people with dementia, five students on placement and a very able teacher. I then felt a desire to tell my own story in greater depth, and did this through the book *Walk the Walk, Talk the Talk*. However, I do see life stories as being a journey with lots of other people, and I was fortunate that 72 friends and family readily agreed to contribute to my story within that book.

How did the idea of writing a new book come about?
I wanted both the previous two books to raise money for dementia charities and to give me a platform from which I could engage with readers. This was picked up by Andrew James at Jessica Kingsley Publishers, who in the summer of 2017 invited me to meet with him to discuss a new book project. This came totally out of the blue for me because after *Walk the Walk, Talk the Talk* I didn't envisage myself writing in the near future. We wanted the book to be unique and different to previous publications; at the time I was reading a lot of Alan Bennett's writing and this encouraged me to consider using a diary format for the bulk of this book.

Picking up on this point, why did you choose the genre of diary for your new book?
At the time Andrew contacted me I had almost finished Alan Bennett's *Keeping On Keeping On*, and really enjoyed this book. This followed reading the diaries of Tony Benn, whose command of the English language and philosophy alongside his politics filled me with admiration. I know how hard the planning and writing process is without intensive professional support, so I looked to what resources I had available, and the obvious source was my diaries, journals and extensive notes made over the past seven years. I was also motivated by the thought that, to the best of our knowledge, no one with dementia had attempted this before, which is consistent with my desire to tackle new challenges. I hoped I could thus produce something innovative, original, unique and readable.

What do you see as the purpose of writing this book?
First, to confront a personal challenge. Second, I see the opportunity to focus in greater depth than previously on my journey with dementia in a way that has not been done before. I hope that it will be useful to a wide range of readers, including professionals, people with dementia and carers, but also the general public. Again, following on from the two previous books, I want to help dementia causes, and half of the book royalties will go to Young Dementia UK, a charity close to my heart.

Can you describe the process you used to create this book?
Writing can be a lonely and isolating experience. So first of all, I recruited four or five friends as allies and helpers, namely Lewis, Nicki, April and Liz. From this I produced a plan, and then re-read through many volumes of

diaries, notebooks, files and journals, making notes along the way. I produced a comprehensive timeline listing all the key events I had experienced since 2010, and then began to reflect deeply upon each of them in turn. I wanted all of the words to be mine, which they are. In the case of Lewis, Nicki and Liz, their support is also in typing each of the chapters from a Dictaphone and supporting me at meetings with the publisher; April and Liz were my advisors and first readers alongside Rosemary, my wife. Each of these four friends gave me detailed and constructive feedback on the drafts. Further support during the course of the process was provided by placement students Darshi, Abi and Andrew.

Did revisiting the diary and writing up this book bring back memories or make you remember events that you have forgotten about?
Writing the book was a cathartic experience, and enabled me to revisit what is a narrow but life-changing period of my life. The events are often hazy and occasionally muddled, but by re-reading my journals and diaries at the point of writing there was a greater sense of clarity. One problem I have with dementia is that I cannot sustain or hold onto this. For Rosemary, re-reading the book was almost certainly a more difficult experience. Her coping strategy is different from mine in the sense that she tries to park and forget the difficult days and experiences which we have lived through together, whereas I have tried to learn from, and then confront, them.

Were there instances where your memories and the diary entries seemed to be very different from one another?
Not really. My diary and journals are I think very accurate. I do rely and lean upon them in the way that previously I would have relied on my memory. Occasionally I would check certain events with another person to verify certain facts. It is worth stating that this book is a memoir and not a biography, in that the events are based upon my recall of them. If in doubt, it is my written memories in diary and journal that I trust rather than my flawed mental recall.

What are your thoughts and feelings when writing?
First to make the work as accurate and truthful as possible in a memoir style, and in so doing to make it readable and interesting to the reader. I feel the narrative is very revealing, and consequently, there is a sense of vulnerability and direct openness which I think comes through.

Do you think that writing allows you to express your feelings more, and if so, how?

I think so. In the context of this book diaries are often very personal and private documents. What I'm seeking to do is to open the door to my diary, so that readers don't just get a sense of what happened on that day but how events and people made me feel. This is consistent with all I have said in talks and meetings for the past five or six years, and is very different from my former way of thinking. Consequently, some exchanges are more positive than others, and the resulting emotions stay with me long after recall of the event.

A diary acts as a way of capturing a memory, whereas dementia is a progressive disease that leads to memory loss. Did you consider this contradiction?

Writing a diary and a journal is a discipline, and the need to keep making entries regularly is crucial in order to document events, emotions and responses. There were many days when dementia prevented me from recording things coherently. On other days, there is much greater clarity and I think this comes through within this book. This is one misunderstanding around dementia – that it is linear in its progression and downward in its trajectory. My experience is that whilst overall the movement is down, there are peaks and troughs, and also that dementia is more than simply memory loss, which again I hope this book goes some way to proving.

Have you ever experienced writer's block and how did you deal with it?

Yes I have, and I have adopted two or three approaches to this. I will either go for a walk with my iPad playing familiar music which I find helpful, or in the case of *Welcome to Our World* I did this with a friend who was supporting me, which allowed us to talk through a piece of writing. On other occasions just getting something written down helps diminish the sense of foreboding through looking at a blank page or screen. Finally, it is fair to say that writer's block is something like what I experience on many days in general life, and I hope that is explained further within the book.

Did you ever feel you would be publishing a third book when you received a diagnosis of dementia?

Not at all, I never thought I'd even publish one!

Do you have any advice for readers considering writing their first book?
First, I would suggest that you read widely, including different writing styles and genre, then look out for local courses which teach writing skills. Following on, share your ideas with someone else you trust, and recruit allies and friends who you can share with and confide in. Then go for it!

Who do you think you will dedicate your new book to?
My previous works have been dedicated to Rosemary, and specific chapters to specific people who were significant in that part of the story. This time I intend the book to be dedicated to all those people who live with young onset dementia, either with a diagnosis or who share their lives with us.

2nd December 2018

Dear clinical psychologist, researcher and commissioner

'Give me...I will'

Give me myself and I will be me

Give me an ear and I will speak

Give me patience and I will relax

Give me music and my heart will dance

Give me joy and I will laugh

Give me a way and I will follow

Give me a baton and I will share

Give me inspiration and I will excel

Give me teaching and I will learn

Give me truth and I will consider

Give me compassion and I will care

Give me identity and I will shine

Give me attachment and I will engage

Give me occupation and I will be focused

Give me inclusion and I will belong

Give me comfort and I will feel warmth

Give me love and I will thrive

There's the evidence, please do something with it now!

Thank you
Your 'professional friend'

Keith

Acronyms and abbreviations

ABA – Achieving Better Access (links to the Expert Reference Group)

ADI – Alzheimer's Disease International

AGM – Annual general meeting

ALWAYS group – Action on Living Well: Asking You

BAFTA – British Academy of Film and Television Arts

BBC – British Broadcasting Corporation

BFI – British Film Institute

BPS – British Psychological Society

CBT – Cognitive behavioural therapy

CEO – Chief executive officer

CFT – Compassion-focused therapy

CIDS – Cognitive Impairment and Dementia Service, West Middlesex Hospital, Hounslow, UK

CQC – Care Quality Commission

CRPD – United Nations Convention on the Rights of Persons with Disabilities

CRUK – Cancer Research UK

DAA – Dementia Action Alliance

DEEP – Dementia Engagement and Empowerment Project

EEG – Electroencephalogram

EKIDS – East Kent Independent Dementia Support

ERG – Expert Reference Group

EU – European Union

FPOP – Faculty of the Psychology of Older People (Faculty of the Division of Clinical Psychology within the BPS)

GAP – Grants Advisory Panel (Alzheimer's Society Research Network)

GP – General practitioner

HR – Human Resources

ICHOM – International Consortium for Health Outcomes Measurement

IDEAL project – Improving the Experience of Dementia and Enhancing Active Life

IPA – Interpretive phenomenological analysis

IT – Information technology

ITV – Independent Television

KMPT – Kent and Medway NHS and Social Care Partnership Trust

LGBT – Lesbian, gay, bisexual, transgender community

MC – Master of Ceremonies

MP – Member of Parliament

MRI scan – Magnetic resonance imaging scan

MSNAP – Memory Services National Accreditation Programme

NHS – National Health Service

NICE – National Institute for Health and Care Excellence

OT – Occupational therapy

PEP team – Primary Excellence Project team

PPI – Public and patient involvement

PREVENT – A large-scale project to examine intervention studies to determine risk factors present in mid-life and thus help prevent dementia

PTFA – Parents, Teachers and Friends Association

Q&A – Questions and answers

RCT – Randomised controlled trial

RSAS – Royal Surgical Aid Society

SATs – Standardised Assessment Tests – at age 11

SENCO – Special educational needs coordinator

SILK – Social Inclusion Living in Kent

SPECAL – Special early care for Alzheimer's: method of understanding dementia linked to the Contented Dementia Trust

SPECT/HMPAO scan – Single photon emission computerised tomography brain scan

SURP – Alzheimer's Society Service User Review Panel

U3A – University of the Third Age

UKDC – UK Dementia Congress

UNISON – Trade union for public sector workers

VALID – Valuing Active Life in Dementia project

VERDe project – Values, Equality, Rights and Dementia

WI – Women's Institute

YDUK – Young Dementia UK charity

YODEL – Young Onset Dementia Engaged Living

Questions for book groups reading Dear Alzheimer's

1. What stood out in this book for you?

2. Before you read this book, what was your experience and perception of dementia, and of people living with dementia?

3. After reading the book, did any of your ideas around dementia change?

4. Which of the challenges that Keith faced stood out to you particularly? Having read the book, what changes do you think could be made to improve everyday experiences for people with dementia?

5. How far do you think a positive mental attitude helps people living with long-term conditions such as dementia? How can you encourage that attitude in your own life, and that of your friends and loved ones?